About the Author

Kathryn Marsden is a nutritionist, freelance health writer and author of several books on healthy eating. Although probably best known for her regular columns in some of the UK's leading magazines and newspapers, and for her best-selling books on food combining and on skin problems, she has long held a special interest in the treatment of digestive disorders and is famous for her informative yet lighthearted lectures on the mysterious rumblings of the gut. She cites genes that made her celebrated uncle a world authority on the history of the flush toilet as the most likely reason behind her whacky sense of humour and her fascination with human plumbing.

Kathryn lives 'among some of the warmest and kindest people on the planet' in the wild west of Scotland, where the air is clear, the water is like wine and yet vegetables are still regarded as a dietary punishment. She believes wholeheartedly in a healthy diet and as much of it organic as possible, but also hopes that she lives by the dictum 'laughter, learned of friends and of gentleness'.

Other Books by Kathryn Marsden

KATHRYN MARSDEN

GOOD GUT
healing

the no-nonsense guide to
bowel & **digestive disorders**

PIATKUS

Copyright © 2003 by Kathryn Marsden

First published in 2003 by
Judy Piatkus (Publishers) Limited
5 Windmill Street
London W1T 2JA
e-mail: info@piatkus.co.uk

The moral right of the author has been asserted

A catalogue record for this book is available from the British Library

Reprinted 2004

ISBN 0 7499 2448 9

Text design and make up by Paul Saunders
Edited by Krystyna Mayer
Technical illustrations by Rodney Paull

This book has been printed on paper manufactured with respect for the environment using wood from managed sustainable resources

Printed and bound in Great Britain by William Clowes Ltd, Beccles, Suffolk

This book is dedicated to my late uncle, Henry Victor Billington, the genuine world authority on the history of the water closet. An ingenious and eccentric wit, exceptional educator and gifted wordsmith, he cheered many an estranged childhood with his outstanding talent and his potty sense of humour, and handed down to his only niece his great love of writing and communication.

The laughter still echoes . . .

I regret to inform you that the nearest W.C. in the district is five miles away. This is rather unfortunate if you are in the habit of going regularly. It may interest you to know that many people take their lunch to make a day of it. By the way, it is built to accommodate 1,000 and it has been decided to replace the old wooden seats . . . to ensure greater comfort especially to those who have to sit a long time . . .

Hoping this will be of use to you and trusting you will be able to go regularly.

From *The Geordie Netty* by Frank Graham (Howe Brothers, Gateshead 1966). This letter was a response to someone enquiring about local toilet facilities. The person replying was, in fact, a church minister who took 'W.C.' to mean 'nearest Wesleyan Chapel'.

Some Notes for Readers

The information that Kathryn includes in her books, articles and lectures has been accumulated from her own personal research and experience and, from the feedback she has received, it would appear to have helped many people. However, it is important that the reader understands that these guidelines are *not* intended to be prescriptive, nor are they an attempt to diagnose or treat any specific condition.

If you are concerned in any way about your health, Kathryn recommends that you visit your own doctor or hospital consultant without delay. She also suggests that you keep your medical adviser informed of any dietary changes you make and of any supplement programmes you intend to follow. Obtain as many details about your condition as possible, asking plenty of questions about any medicines that may be prescribed to you. *Do not* stop taking any currently prescribed medication without first talking to your general practitioner. In the meantime, follow a varied and sensible diet that contains plenty of fresh, unprocessed wholefoods, daily fresh fruits and vegetables, and filtered or bottled water. Take regular exercise and avoid cigarette smoke.

Kathryn regrets that, due to the cost and time involved in dealing with her already overloaded postbag, she can no longer reply individually to letters or comment on specific case histories. She is, however, always delighted to hear from readers and promises to read every letter.

Kathryn's views are completely independent. She is not employed by any pharmaceutical company, supplement supplier or food producer, nor is she persuaded in any way, financially or otherwise, to recommend particular products or services.

Contents

Foreword by Dr Jen W. Tan MB, BS

We do not give our bowels and digestive systems the attention that they deserve.

On the one hand, so-called 'civilised' people with good manners are embarrassed by what the gut does and what it produces. On the other, the medical profession hasn't yet woken up to the important role that the digestive system plays in determining our general health. One may accept that farting is normal. But what are we to make of the importance of examining our faeces for colour and consistency, never mind aroma! However, there is a lot of sense in all of this, as you will see from this book.

Complementary medicine has come a long way in gaining recognition by the orthodoxy – but it still has some distance to go. I come from the orthodox side of the fence, so I understand the problem. When I was a medical student, we were taught that food allergies were limited to coeliac disease and very rare cases of peanut allergy. But no doctor understood the concept of leaky gut syndrome or gut dysbiosis. And while some doctors now acknowledge that the irritable bowel syndrome exists *outside* the mind, few are able to accept the way in which candida in the gut can cause ill-health.

Nevertheless, seeing what can happen to a myriad of diverse symptoms when healthy gut flora is replaced, offending foods are removed from a diet and digestion is improved should make even the most orthodox medical specialist stop and think.

Kathryn Marsden has never avoided the unconventional. Over the years, she has played a significant part in bringing orthodox and complementary medicine closer together with writing that is clear and easily understood by both sides. This book will not only highlight the importance of the gut to those suffering ill-health, but will also bring to the attention of the medical profession concepts they only hear of from their patients.

Dr Jen W. Tan MB, BS

Foreword by Sarah Stacey

Once again, Kathryn Marsden has produced a must-read book, which should be on everyone's bookshelf. The unromantic but hugely common problems of the gut have been a taboo for too long. In her usual direct and chatty style, Kathryn breaks through the barriers to give a brilliantly clear account of the possible problems and how to deal with them. Many of the solutions are simple lifestyle shifts to do with diet and there are comprehensive directions on using natural products. This book makes it clear that you don't need to suffer in the way so many people take for granted. Please buy it now for the sake of your health and happiness.

Sarah Stacey
Wellbeing Editor, *YOU* magazine
Vice President of the Guild of Health Writers UK

Acknowledgements

A trillion times thanks to my posse of proofreaders, Sarah Stacey, Michael Burke, Helen Dick, Georgina Bond and Dr Jen Tan for their constructive and oh so sensible input. Endless appreciation to Georgina for her cover copy and to Sarah for her gifted and awe-inspiring editor's pen.

To naturopaths Kerrin Booth and Jayne Tancred for their practitioner expertise, and likewise to nutritionist Alison Cullen who dealt so patiently with my many questions.

A very special thank you to Gillian Hamer for her guidance, wisdom and support throughout the project.

Again to Dr Jen Tan and to Sarah Stacey for writing the forewords.

To Paul Saunders for his *always* excellent design.

To Anna Crago for never saying 'Oh no, not you again!' – and for lending her terrific sense of humour to the potentially fractious and fatiguing task of checking the manuscript.

To Michael Alcock, for his encouragement and for being my very special agent.

And most especially – and for the rest of my days – to my husband Richard, for never tiring of listening to my ideas, for his lateral thinking, for the brainstorming when I got stuck, for taking the domestic strain completely on his shoulders while I researched and wrote and for the imagination that eventually gave birth to the title.

I would never have made it without you.

There is an old proverb that tells of a man who was shown what hell looked like. He was taken to a room where a group of people sat around a huge pot of stew. They each held a long-handled spoon that reached the pot but which was too long and awkward to turn round to reach their mouths. Everyone was hollow-eyed, emaciated and desperate.

Then the man was taken and shown heaven. The room was the same, the stew pot was the same, the spoons were the same. But the people were well nourished, happy and full of joy and laughter. The man shook his head in wonder. 'I don't understand,' he said, 'what's going on? Everything appears to be as it was in the other place but these people look so well.'

'Look again,' suggested his guide. 'Don't you see? Here they have learned to feed each other.'

1.

Introductory Rumblings

❝ Here, at whatever hour you come, you will find light and help and human kindness. ❞

Inscription under the lamp outside the hospital of humanitarian theologian and missionary Dr Albert Schweitzer, at Lambaréné, Gabon in Africa.

What do you do if your digestive system plays you up on a daily basis, disrupting your day or disturbing your night? If you continually need to watch what you eat, if you suffer regular 'repeating' bloating or nausea, if your bowel movements are either far too frequent or singularly scarce, your stomach churns constantly and unpleasantly or you cannot remember ever *not* being windy? Who do you talk to if you're plagued with an irritable bowel, acid reflux or diverticulitis? How do you cope with agonising haemorrhoids (piles) or a smarting hiatus hernia? How would you know if you were suffering from leaky gut syndrome, or an overgrowth of yeast or parasites? What happens if you simply don't know why you're feeling miserably uncomfortable? Where do you turn if your digestive system is simply *dysfunctional*?

Well, you've come to the right place – although can I say, here and now, if you find that words such as faeces, flatus or farting offend your sensibilities, then this book is definitely not for you. However, if you're suffering any kind of bloating, indigestion, food sensitivity, acid reflux, digestive discomfort or bad-tempered bowel, then I do implore you to read on, not only because *Good Gut Healing* has a lot of seriously sensible information that could be helpful to you, but also because it should raise a smile or two.

Apart from the fact that it's much quoted as the best medicine, laughter is also said to be the most civilised music in the world. When we laugh about something, we're less likely to be stressed, more likely to relax and far more inclined to remember the information. So, as you make your way through the chapters, my hope is that the irreverent, down-to-earth approach will not only engender a giggle or two here and there, but will also help you to feel very much better. And that's the essence of this book. *Practical information wrapped in plain straightforward language and tied up with humour.*

This is a book that I've always intended to write. It's been on my mind for years but, for one reason or another, and in no particular order, other projects, other books, the results of a nasty accident that slowed me down a bit, bereavement, remarriage, family, patients and teaching always took up my time.

But the subject lingered. Gut gripes are distressingly common. Questions about all manner of disorders to do with crabby colons, snarling stomachs and testy dyspepsia have always been at the top of my stack of incoming mail. And it's a digestive fact of life that if the gut isn't healthy, then neither is the rest of the body.

Unfortunately, no one apart from medics and health practitioners much likes to use the word 'gut'. At best, it reminds people of fishing rods or surgical stitches. At worst, it conjures a picture we'd probably rather not have of that ignored, neglected and rejected colonic cloister; in other words – our extremely unattractive intestines. Say 'digestive system' and most of us think 'stomach'. Say 'bowels', and thoughts descend to waste products, bacteria and unpleasant smells. Doctors call it the gastro-intestinal tract, which they shorten to g.i. tract. But the word 'gut' is, and will always be, the colloquy that most closely and accurately describes the full length of the mouth-to-anus inner tube that runs from the top, quite literally, to the bottom of every human being. So, like it or not, 'gut' it is.

The good news is that, in most cases, the common conditions that affect the gut are not difficult to treat. During my clinic work as a nutritionist, improving the comfort and behaviour of the 'bowel and burp departments' is something with which I had particular success. I've also developed a bit of a reputation (never quite decided if this is a good or a bad thing) for injecting humour into my lectures on gut disorders. Well, without a few belly laughs, the digestive system could be just a bit boring, don't you think?

At one college where, for many years, I took weekend classes of adult students for Basic Nutrition and Healthy Eating, the Course Director used to joke that no one would have difficulty locating the room that held my group. No, we weren't all farting. But we did spend much of each day convulsed in guffawing giggles. No wonder anyone looking for my room was told 'Hear that laughter? Just follow it.' We had a lot of fun, but the interesting point for me is that students say they remembered the lectures because they were allowed to lighten up and laugh.

So, no prizes for guessing that the digestive tract in general – and the large intestine in particular – are favourite subjects of mine. To some, they might seem odd choices. After all, these are topics that few people seem happy – or feel relaxed enough about – to discuss in private, never mind in public. I think we already agree; the gut is a pretty repulsive piece of anatomy. Slimy and smelly, and to borrow the name of a Hogwart's House, slytherin. 'In brief, the gut is despicable and reptilian, not at all like the brain from which wise thoughts emerge. Clearly, the gut is an organ only a scientist would love.'[1] Or, in my case, a nutritionist. Or, if you've reached this far in my introduction to *Good Gut Healing*, I imagine you must be interested, too, if not in what your gut looks like or how it behaves, then in why it isn't working as it should.

There's an old maxim that says disease – and death – begin in the colon. And another that believes 'we are what we eat'. Both sayings are oh so true and apply to anyone who doesn't absorb nutrients properly from their food, passes food that is only partially digested or finds it difficult to pass anything at all. Essentially, then, we are what we crap – or don't crap. And yet most of us are too shy to talk about this most natural of all functions, even when we suspect that there might be something wrong.

We may laugh, in private and in company, at 'toilet humour' but are often too self-conscious to discuss the subject at a serious level. From the flatulence of Johnny Fartpants to breaking wind in the film *Blazing Saddles*, we delight in laughing at someone else's faux pas but can feel humiliated and distressed if we're the 'guilty party'. I know one elderly gent who always blames his dog, another one (not so elderly) who punctuates every conversation with burps and a lady of indeterminable age who simply 'whoopee cushions' her way through life as if everyone else was deaf.

In fact, low-level digestive rumblings and flatulent emissions are totally, utterly, absolutely and completely natural! In some countries, a

1. *The Second Brain*, Michael Gershon, HarperPerennial 1999, page xi.

jolly good belch is a compliment to the host for a fine meal – although I did hear recently that, in one town in America, it's illegal to belch without a doctor's certificate! Let's be honest: only the chosen few can eat beans without passing wind and begging someone's pardon one way or another.

We've all suffered at one time or another from gas, trapped wind, indigestion, cramps, constipation or diarrhoea, perhaps as a result of eating too late, drinking or eating to excess, or picking up a food-borne bug. We shouldn't be surprised. Morning, noon and night, throughout life, we push whatever we fancy into our mouths and down our gullets with little or no thought for what happens to it once it's out of sight. We hardly ever chew food properly (who do you know who doesn't rush their meals?), and then we expect our long-suffering digestive systems to mash it all up, utilise the good, discard the bad, kill off any unwanted bugs, stay quiet, never complain and never go wrong.

When they do grumble, out come the indigestion remedies and the annoying symptoms are usually knocked out with never a thought to the consequences . . . until the next time!

If symptoms persist, your first port of call is likely to be your doctor. This is a very sensible move, since examination and discussion can be vital to early diagnosis and successful treatment. It's much better to visit the doctor and find nothing seriously wrong than to wait until it's too late to do anything. In most cases, all that may be required is a check-up and some reassurance; both are important parts of health care. Sometimes, a prescription for just the right medication can despatch the problem in a matter of days or weeks.

But what if the medication doesn't suit you or simply doesn't work? Or if it works while you're taking it but the condition starts again when you stop the treatment? Is there anything that can be done to reduce the risk of a recurrence that doesn't involve a life of perpetual discomfort or prescription drugs? What if, happily, your complaint isn't life-threatening but, unhappily, is not just an isolated episode of digestive distress? It could be that tests show nothing is wrong and yet the symptoms remain. Is there something else you could try?

Yes, there is. You can try a different approach to everyday eating, simple lifestyle changes, and the sensible use of tried and tested herbal medicines, healing foods and other gentle therapies. Or, in some cases, once the medical prescription has dealt with the severest symptoms, more natural treatments can take over to restore inner strength and resistance. And when they do, we may wonder why we never tried them before.

Did you know, for example, that it used to be common practice for all medics to prescribe routinely those less intrusive treatments such as detox, fasting, reflexology, hydrotherapy, manipulation of bones, massage, herbal medicine or food therapy? They fell from favour only when the introduction of chemical extracts and synthetic drugs began to take over at around the turn of the twentieth century. Sadly, many of these ancient remedies, although effective and still available, tend to be dismissed as worthless or considered only when everything else fails.

Nothing, of course, is a cure-all. There is no diet, no pill, no potion to eradicate every ill – no 'one size fits all'. When it comes to nutritional therapy, there is only one rule and that is that we should ignore the rules and treat everyone as an individual. That's because there are, around the world, as many beneficial diets and ways of eating healthily as there are races, creeds, colours and personalities. What suits one person may not suit another, nor is it meant to. Nevertheless, there is still a great deal of dietary and other information well worth following; advice that is known to relieve symptoms, regulate imbalances and enhance well-being.

What's included in the book

1. The Inside Story

After my initial 'rumblings', the first thing you'll come across is a journey through the digestive system; quite literally, the inside story. I hope you won't dismiss it as boring anatomy or something you're sure cannot possibly be of interest because this is stuff I think you'll be really glad you picked up on. There's nothing heavy here. It's simply a light-hearted trip in the company of an ordinary meal, describing some of the things that can go wrong if the gut isn't functioning as it should. You'll find out why our insides are so prone to disruption, why a discontented colon or a sore stomach can be the beginnings of disease, and what you can do to reduce the risk of these problems happening.

2. Going Through the Motions

I hope that this section will encourage everyone who reads it to take more interest in their waste products.

3. How Long Does it Take?

The movement of food from one end of the body to the other will vary enormously from person to person but the *longer* the transit time, the *greater* the risk of a number of bowel diseases including constipation, diverticulosis and cancer of the colon. This section looks at transit time and what you can do to speed things up.

4. Where Does it Hurt?

Tips on how to communicate with your GP.

5. What's Up?

Suffering from a particular condition or know someone else who is trying to find information? This section explains what's behind a whole range of different gut gripes, from acid reflux, bloating, constipation and candida, down past irritable bowel syndrome and all the way to ulcers. If you already have a definite diagnosis, you can turn straight to the problem. If you're not sure, you can learn more by reading through each condition and finding out which symptoms, if any, apply.

Towards the end of each main section, you'll find an *action plan* that includes dietary advice, lifestyle changes and remedies to help you to feel more comfortable and reduce the risk of recurrence. I'll tell you which foods can be helpful and those that may make symptoms worse, and where to find more information. Each section also has a quick ten-point point reminder detailing the most important moves you can make now.

6. If You Do Nothing Else . . .

These pages are the fast-track for those of you who are too busy just at the moment to read the whole book but who need immediate help. So, if you do nothing else, at least read this section.

7. Essential Extras

This part of the book does exactly what it says on the tin, providing you with essential extra information on:

- How to recognise which foods could be potential gut wrenchers and which foods are most likely to be soothing and healing.

- New shopping strategies that help you to improve the quality of your diet by swapping the bad and the not so good for the much better.

- How to gain the best from the food that you eat, take the strain off your overworked digestive system and nurture it to work more efficiently.

- Which dietary fibres really work and which ones could be making matters worse.

- The 'liquid news'. Why fluid intake is so vital, which drinks are best and which ones may be best avoided.

- The benefits of friendly gut flora. Why good bugs are beneficial – in fact, essential – to your long-term health.

- Why stress can have a seriously damaging effect on the digestive system and what you can do to ease the strain.

- How simple food combining can be a positive step forward for certain disorders of the digestion and bowel.

Signs, symbols, hints and tips

Throughout the book, you'll come across boxes, symbols and signs that alert you to special information:

 Did you know?
The big question mark has bites of info that should help to add to your understanding.

 VERY IMPORTANT POINT
An exclamation mark indicates **a very important point** that I think you should be aware of.

 In more detail . . .
Technical stuff that isn't essential reading but that could extend your knowledge about a particular condition or remedy.

WWW **Web links** to the Internet for interesting sites and more information.

Helpful hint
Foods or actions that can be a major help towards easing a particular digestive discomfort.

 Beware
Foods or actions that are known to aggravate a particular condition.

Jargon buster

This is where you'll find easy-to-follow explanations for those sometimes baffling words or phrases.

KATHRYN'S TOP TEN TIPS
The reminder boxes at the ends of sections will help you to remember those really important bits of information.

For more information
The double arrow refers you to other parts of the book that may be especially relevant. For example:

For more information on irritable bowel syndrome see page 195. For more information on acid reflux see page 36.

 Snippets
The scissor sign indicates snippets of information that don't seem to fit anywhere else but that I thought you might find interesting or fun.

What's *not* included

At the planning stages of this book, I made the decision to cover the listed conditions in some detail and not to try to be all things to all people. The conditions were chosen on the basis of being the gut disorders most commonly presented during my years in nutrition practice. I have therefore *not* included acute (short-term) illnesses such as food poisoning or infectious diarrhoea. Nor do I talk about inflammatory bowel diseases such as

Crohn's disease or ulcerative colitis, coeliac disease, diseases of the liver or pancreas, or colon cancer. These are serious conditions that, I believe, warrant much more space than is available here.

I hope that the information I've gathered and included in *Good Gut Healing* will give you plenty of self-help and lots of answers to any questions you might have. Some recommendations you may be aware of, but many others will be new to you. All are well worth considering.

In the meantime, I wish you laughter, the love of friends and, without delay, the very best of better health.

Kathryn Marsden

Kathryn

Author's note

The human digestive system is so complicated and so very clever that even the most highly qualified specialists will admit that they still don't understand all of its idiosyncrasies. I am merely a nutritionist and health writer who enjoys a passionate interest in all workings of the gastrointestinal tract and who has attempted here to share that fascination with you. I've spent many months researching and checking the information included in *Good Gut Healing* and hope that it is as accurate as is humanly possible. Please understand, however, that the material is *not* intended to be prescriptive, nor does it attempt to diagnose or treat any specific condition or replace medical advice.

2.

The Inside Story

❝ Definition of *Diaphragm*, n. A muscular partition separating disorders of the chest from disorders of the bowels. ❞

The Devil's Dictionary, Ambrose Gwinett Bierce, 1842–*c.* 1914

Both digestion and absorption are as essential to our survival as breathing. That's why understanding what's happening to food once it's been eaten is an important step towards good gut healing. You can skip to page 23 if you like but I think this is valuable information for you to know, so I hope you'll stay with me.

First, let's look at what goes on in a healthy digestion. Then, as we progress through the book, we'll see what help is available for some of the common conditions that can occur when the system doesn't work quite as well as it should.

In a nutshell

One easy way to picture the gastrointestinal tract – the food-processing pipe that runs through the body from one end to the other – is as a kind of extended ring doughnut. If you think of the doughnut hole as the space within the gut wall, you can see that it is, in fact, part of the outside world, even though it's inside the body.

Dr Michael Gershon says in his book *The Second Brain*: 'The design of the body can be understood by paraphrasing T.S. Eliot. We are indeed hollow men and, although Eliot did not say it (he was a sexist pig), also hollow women.'

Once we grasp the idea of this 'hollowness', it makes it easier to understand that food isn't truly *inside* the body until it's been absorbed through the gut wall.

And here's the reason why our 'inside skin' is constructed so differently from our 'outside skin'. Instead of being tough and impenetrable, protecting us from our external environment, the gut wall has to be permeable, so that nutrients from our food supply can move through it. The problem for so many of us, though, is that quite of lot of our food *isn't* properly digested or absorbed.

Jargon buster

Digestion is the process by which large and complex food substances are broken down into smaller, simpler units ready for absorption.

Absorption is the process by which these nutrients cross the gut wall into the blood and lymph circulation and are then transported throughout the body to all of the cells, where they are used for a variety of activities.

The role of the GI tract

The main purpose of your gastrointestinal tract is to:

- Digest your food.
- Break that food down into particles small enough to be absorbed via the bloodstream into the cells.
- Convert nutrients into energy.
- Act as a first-line defence against infection.
- Detoxify chemicals and other waste products.
- Remove wastes from the body.

So once you've eaten, that's it – or is it?

Once you've finished a meal, you probably don't give it another thought but, for the food, this is just the beginning of a journey of labyrinthine proportions.

Let's begin at the beginning

It doesn't occur to most people that digestion occurs in the mouth. But that's where it kicks off.

When we put food into our mouths, nature's plan is that we are supposed to chew thoroughly, using our teeth to split each bite into smaller particles. Sadly, most of us eat far too quickly, gulping as we go and hardly giving our meals a chance at proper digestion.

Chewing is not simply to make swallowing easier. As we masticate, saliva lubricates the food, and a digestive enzyme in the saliva begins to break down starchy foods.

Chewing also helps to demolish the undigestible fibrous parts (cellulose membranes) of fruits, salad foods and raw vegetables. Without this action, our bodies wouldn't be able to get hold of the vital vitamins, minerals and other nutrients in these essential fresh foods.

Jargon buster

Amylase is the enzyme in saliva that splits complex carbohydrates (also sometimes called complex starches) such as bread, pasta and rice into smaller components ready for more complete digestion further down the digestive tract.

Did you know?
Ever wondered why we so often feel the urge to defaecate immediately after a meal? The action of chewing sends signals to the stomach to 'get ready, there's food on the way', and to the bowel, warning it to empty to make room for a new delivery of wastes.

You chew proteins, too

Even though protein foods such as meat, poultry, eggs, nuts, soya protein, cheese and fish are not *chemically* digested in the mouth, they still need to be mashed up by the teeth, making them ready for further disintegration later on in the process. Swallowing proteins in larger pieces simply means that, however hard the stomach juices work to break it up, some of that protein will probably stay undigested.

In more detail . . .
Note that salivary enzymes help to break down *starchy* foods, not pro-teins. Saliva is known, chemically, as an alkaline substance – the opposite of acid – and cannot dissolve proteins. Apart from the fact that the membranes of our mouth and tongue are not designed to withstand strong acids, if saliva were acidic, our teeth would crumble and fall out.

Once food has been chewed, it is pushed by the tongue to the back of the mouth, where it slips down the gullet.

What can go wrong?

- Lazy chewing means that saliva doesn't lubricate the food, leaving it dryer and more difficult to swallow than it should be. It can 'catch' in the gullet, causing the unpleasant sensation of something being 'stuck' in the upper chest area, which will only be cleared when information from the enteric nervous system (ENS, or 'bowel brain', see page 199) triggers reflexes to dislodge the food and propel it downwards. This scenario is not likely to be fatal and is not the same as the life-threatening choking caused if food blocks the windpipe. Adequate chewing does, however, also reduce the risk of choking. Everyone should learn how to carry out the recommended first aid for this emer-gency, the Heimlich manoeuvre, which aims to dislodge airway ob-struction using a forceful and sudden upwards compression of the upper abdomen in the centre 'V' shape below the ribs.

- Even when swallowing seems easy, if we don't masticate every mouthful properly food isn't broken down into small enough particles, thus putting greater strain on the next stages of digestion. Poor chew-ing results in enzymes in the saliva not being distributed evenly through the food.

- It's likely that rushing your meal will cause you to burp, bloat up, fart or suffer digestive discomfort.

- If digestion doesn't go according to plan, even at this early stage in the process, it's probable that you won't fully digest your meal or absorb all the available nourishment from it. What a waste.

When we swallow . . .

. . . our food passes from the mouth, down into the first part of the digestive tract, called the gullet or oesophagus (say 'essoffagus'). Think of it as a lift shaft.

Muscular squeezing of the gullet allows the food to travel at a regulated speed down this pipe, each mouthful taking anything from three to ten seconds to make the journey. This is so your grub doesn't crash straight into your stomach. At the bottom of the lift shaft, there's a 'door' (known as the lower oesophageal sphinctre or LES) that opens into the stomach with a one-way valve that is designed to help prevent food from coming back up the other way.

Jargon buster

The **lower oesophageal sphinctre** is the 'door' between your gullet and your stomach. Remembering what it does could be important if you suffer from acid reflux or hiatus hernia. We'll look again at this problem later on.

?

Did you know?
The one-way valve does become two-way if you need to be sick. The stomach contracts and the doorway opens to propel unwanted contents upwards, allowing the body to get rid of the potentially poisonous debris.

Next stop, the stomach

The stomach is not, as many people mistakenly believe, in the belly. The area below your belt contains your small and large intestines. Your stomach is further up. Pinpoint yours by looking down at the left front of your body and imagining a J-shaped sac filling most of the space from just below the *left* nipple diagonally across to just above the navel or centre of the waistband.

Your stomach performs three main functions.

1. It acts as a storage container for meals, controlling the transit of food through the system. Without this 'way station' food would be dumped straight into the small intestine. Indeed, 'dumping syndrome' is a common problem for people who have had their stomachs surgically removed.

2. It produces gastric juices:
   - **Hydrochloric acid** destroys some of the potentially hazardous contaminants that might be in our food, such as bacteria and other micro-organisms.
   - **Pepsin**, an enzyme begins processing proteins.
   - **Lipase**, another enzyme, starts sorting out the fats.

3. It churns your meals around, reducing food to a semi-liquid state so that it's ready to be passed on – a little at a time – into the next department. Your stomach actually tumbles everything around approximately every twenty seconds, allowing the stored food to come into contact with those gastric juices I mentioned above.

Did you know?
Hydrochloric acid is so strong and corrosive that it can dissolve iron filings. The reason the stomach doesn't digest itself and the stomach wall doesn't get burned by acid is because it's protected by a thick layer of mucus.

What can go wrong?

- If the stomach lining gets irritated by such things as too much highly spiced food, alcohol or smoking, or by non-steroidal anti-inflammatory drugs (NSAIDs, usually prescribed for arthritis), the condition is known as gastritis – literally, inflammation of the gastric lining. Symptoms may include nausea, indigestion and pain in the upper chest.

- Although it's not always correctly diagnosed, *lack* of gastric acid can be just as common as *over*-acidity. Reduced levels of hydrochloric acid result in a condition known as hypochlorhydria; when there is no hydrochloric acid at all, it's called achlorhydria. Either situation will lead to an incomplete digestion of proteins, which itself can create a number of health problems. But what's also interesting is that the many symptoms of low gastric acid – heartburn, bloating, belching, nausea, upper chest discomfort – are exactly like those of excess acid. Other common signs of there being not enough hydrochloric acid include sensitivity to certain foods, symptoms associated with candidiasis, parasites and disturbed gut flora, anal irritation, passing undigested food in the stools, peeling or ridged nails and skin problems – especially acne or red blotches on the cheeks or nose.

- If bacteria known as *Helicobacter pylori* are allowed to multiply in the stomach, the likely consequence could be a gastric ulcer.

- Any weakness of the oesophageal valve or of the muscles in the diaphragm can allow an upper part of the stomach wall and the lowest part of the oesophageal tube to 'slip up' into the chest cavity. Known as a 'sliding' hiatus hernia (see page 167), upward pressure caused by the weakness pushes acid through the opening – hence the feeling of heartburn, or acid reflux, when food is able to backflow into the gullet.

Did you know?
Anything that ends with 'itis' nearly always indicates a condition associated with inflammation.

For more information on ulcers see page 235. For more information on acid reflux and heartburn see page 36. For more information on hiatus hernia see page 167.

From the stomach . . .

. . . the liquidised food is pushed slowly downwards through another doorway at the bottom end of the stomach, called the pyloric sphincter, into the next section of tube, the small intestine, which is an amazingly complex 6 metres (just over 20 feet) of miracle conduit.

Jargon buster

The small intestine, sometimes also referred to as the small colon or small bowel, has three important sections. The first port of call after the stomach is called the **duodenum**. Only 30 centimetres (12 inches) in length, it's here that most of the minerals from our food are absorbed. Next comes the 2.4-metre/8-foot-long **jejenum**, which deals with water-soluble vitamins, carbohydrates and proteins. The third and longest section is the **ileum** – 3.6 metres (12 feet) of tubing responsible for fats, fat-soluble vitamins, cholesterol and bile salts. You don't need to remember these names. Just think of it all as a busy street with lots of twists and turns, and different doorways or ducts that secrete a variety of substances from accessory glands along the way, including the pancreas and the gall bladder.

The acid/alkali balance in the duodenum is critical. The acidic contents from the stomach trigger the release of bile and bile salts (soapy stuff) squeezed out into the street from the gall bladder to help emulsify any fat in the food. It's a bit like putting washing-up liquid into greasy water. (Bile also acts like a natural 'disinfectant' and encourages the accumulation of good bacteria.)

It's worth pointing out here that this first section of the small intestine doesn't have the protective lining of the stomach wall that prevents it from being damaged by acids. So the body has a set of very clever hormones that can sense how much acid is likely to be coming by and how much alkali is needed. It relays this information to the pancreas which, in addition to enzymes, also produces natural bicarbonates (think of baking soda) that neutralise the acid. This balancing act is vital because pancreatic (digestive) enzymes will only digest our food if the pH is neutral or slightly alkaline; they're destroyed if the area remains acidic.

Jargon buster

pH is the symbol used to indicate the acidity or alkalinity of a substance. It works on a scale of 1 to 14, with 1 being very acid and 14 being very alkaline. Neutral (neither one nor the other) is 7. The most familiar use of pH to most of us is in the labelling on skin-care products, where 'pH balanced' means that the product matches the slightly acid mantle of the skin, which is between 5 and 5.6.

There are three important enzymes. One called protease deals with proteins, amylase (which you remember is also found in saliva) breaks complex carbohydrates (starches) down into simple sugars, and lipase works with bile to digest fats. All along the street, other microscopically tiny doorways open up, pulling nutrients into the bloodstream.

A particularly essential 'department' with important connections to the small intestine is the liver. This massive detoxification plant filters and deactivates many of the undesirable substances that we take in with our food, water and medications. It produces a constant flow of bile which, as well as being used to help in the breakdown of fats, assists the detoxification process by carrying unwanted residues of drugs, hormones, pesticides and other chemicals out of the body.

The pancreas, too, is a busy little gland with more than one job. Apart from all those digestive enzymes and acid supressors, it's responsible for producing hormones (insulin and glucagon) that regulate the blood sugar levels.

What can go wrong?

- Anything that upsets digestive secretions or damages the lining of the small intestine can have serious repercussions for our long-term health.

- The first part of the small intestine, the duodenum, can become ulcerated, just like the stomach.

- If bile doesn't flow freely, not only the liver and gall bladder could be in trouble. Bad bacteria and toxins build up and fats don't get digested. Bloating, flatulence, indigestion, allergies, headaches and constipation are just a few of the signs of poor liver function. If bile becomes too concentrated, gallstones are the likely result. A blocked bile duct causes pressure that requires immediate surgical attention.

For more information on gallstones see page 135.

- If the pancreas isn't producing the right quantity of enzymes, or the enzymes get destroyed, digestion can be severely impaired. Mild but persistent pancreatic insufficiency is believed to be quite common. Signs include abdominal discomfort, indigestion, gas and wastes that contain undigested matter. Pancreatic enzymes, like the bile, help to bump off bacteria and stop them creeping into places where they might be harmful. In particular, protein-digesting enzymes (pro-teases), are in charge of destroying other unwanted micro-organisms, yeasts, parasites and protozoa. If bad bugs take hold, they feed off your food supply, steal nourishment from you, and cause undigested food to decompose. Result? Decay, toxicity and some very bad odours. You could be at greater risk of allergies, candidiasis and infection, leading to a compromised immune system.

- In turn, irritation and inflammation of the sensitive surfaces of the small intestine by yeasts or particles of undigested food can lead to leaky gut syndrome, in which the tiny 'perforations' become damaged or eroded; larger molecules of undigested food leak into the blood-stream, upsetting the immune system, increasing the risk of allergic reactions and hindering the absorption of all that really vital nourish-ment. Other conditions linked to inflammation and malabsorption of nutrients in the small intestine include coeliac disease (gluten intoler-ance) and inflammatory bowel diseases such as ulcerative colitis and Crohn's disease.

For more information on leaky gut syndrome see page 222.

In more detail . . .

Back where we were a moment ago, at the end of the small intestine, is yet another valve that allows the flow of liquid wastes and other matter into the large intestine but stops it going back again. It's called the ileo-caecal (say 'illeeo-seecal') valve. This name makes sense, as it's the junction between the last part of the small intestine called the ileum and the beginning of the large intestine called the caecum.

Helpful hint

The ileo-caecal valve is down on the right-hand side of the body, just above where your abdomen reaches your right hip bone. I'm telling you about this because knowing where it's located could be helpful later in the book. On page 78 there is a very simple massage technique you can do for yourself that could help reduce a number of unpleasant symptoms. So stay tuned if you have candidiasis, constipation, irritable bowel syndrome or diverticular disease.

Now we've reached the large intestine

Also called the large colon or large bowel, it's responsible for the absorption of electrolytes (salts) and water, and for the sorting out and storage of waste products. It's called 'large' not because of its length – at 1.7 metres (5 feet) it's actually only one-third of the length of the small intestine – but because of its chunky diameter. It includes the rectum (the last 13 centimetres/5 inches) and anus (the hole at the bottom).

Jargon buster

In case you were wondering . . . The word **bowel** is a derivation from the Latin *botulus*, and the French word boel, meaning 'sausage'. And that's just what the large – and the small – intestines look like. A load of long, linked, much-folded sausages.

Efficient elimination of wastes is just as important to your health as digestion itself, and much serious disease could be avoided if we all paid more heed to the messages we get from our bowels.

By the time the digested food reaches this part of the body, all the essential nutrients have been absorbed. All that's left is a load of mush that needs processing ready for exit. Along the way, as water is reabsorbed, it turns to semi-mush; by the time it reaches the rectum, it has squelched itself into soft but fully formed faeces. In the course of a day, the colon reabsorbs around 1½ litres (2½ pints) of water. Most people don't ever drink that much fluid and then wonder why they're constipated.

Billions of bacteria, some friendly, some not so nice, get involved around about here. B vitamins and vitamin K are manufactured. And, of course, a fair amount of gas is produced in the process.

As all this is going on, the muscular movement of those all-important pockets churns and mix the wastes, and waves of peristaltic contractions propel it all along and eventually south or, if you're reading this in Australia or the Falkland Islands, north. Eventually, the solids end up in the rectum, waiting for the call to be ejected, and then the muscular movement pushes the faeces towards the outside world. When the need to defacate occurs, you're finally in control.

What can go wrong?

- Lack of fluid in the diet leaves the wastes too dry. They travel more slowly and become difficult to pass.

- Lack of dietary fibre means that waste doesn't bulk up and, again, is more difficult to pass from one pocket to the next. The likely consequence is constipation.

- Poor muscle tone, usually a result of lack of exercise and ageing, can cause crap to procrastinate and shrivel into hard, pellet-like stools.

- Constipation and straining can lead to haemorrhoids, also called piles. These swollen veins are a common cause of rectal bleeding, irritation and general misery.

- Faeces that hang around in the colon for too long not only putrefy or 'go off', but also produce some very nasty toxins which may be reabsorbed into the bloodstream.

- Slow transit can cause diverticular disease or diverticulosis (referred to as diverticulitis if the diverticula pouches in the intestinal wall become inflamed). This is common in the elderly but can affect younger people, too. Low-fibre diets, lack of fluid intake, poor digestion and constipation are all contributing factors.

- Long-term unresolved constipation is associated with an increased risk of colon cancer.

- Stress and anxiety can disturb the natural rhythm and workings of all of the digestive system and, especially, the large intestine, increasing the risk of irritable bowel syndrome.

Recommended reading

The Second Brain by Dr Michael Gershon is the story behind the discovery of the enteric nervous system, or ENS, the body's 'second brain'. It's now proven that it's the ENS, or 'bowel brain', and not the brain in our head that controls our bowel function. This is a fascinating read, if a bit technical in places, and I'd highly recommend it to anyone who suffers from any kind of digestive or bowel disorder and most especially if you're stricken with irritable bowel syndrome.

3.

Going Through the Motions

> ❝ Politicians and diapers [nappies] have one thing in common. They should both be changed regularly and for the same reason. ❞
>
> Anon

Even though many people remain as reluctant as ever to examine or discuss their waste products, such observations can be a useful guide to inner and outer health. The Brits, especially, have a long history of unwillingness to even think about that most normal of all activities. It was different in Roman times. Lavatories were communal: rows of bum-shaped holes where folks farted in unison and discussed the day's events with ne'er a hint of embarrassment. You may feel that this is going a bit too far but if you're not going at all, might I suggest that you loosen up a little and read on?

Around the globe, attitudes differ. Many European lavatories are designed with a collecting platform – a kind of 'continental shelf' installed so that you can see what you've done. Many more are contrived to be used in the entirely natural squat position so that you can actually see what you're doing while you're doing it.

Unfortunately for the rest of the so-called civilised world, the 'sit-up' flush toilet is probably the worst design for viewing our excreta in any detail or for encouraging regular, relaxed motions. Could this be why so many bathrooms or conveniences in the Western hemisphere resemble the back room of an untidy newsagent's shop, with books, papers and magazines stacked in accessible heaps to relieve the boredom for those who are either caught between two stools or haven't got around to passing any at all?

It's no use brushing bowel habits under the loo mat

It's well known that having the courage to examine your own stools could, seriously, save your life, so it's important to pay attention. If you don't know what colour it is, have no idea of its shape or size, whether it floats or sinks or if it flushes away first time, you're not concentrating. There's no need to poke it about but do please check the paper or the pan at least once a week. The designer detail of your waste products can give you a valuable guide to your general health.

If you're dropping grapeshot, nuts or anything that sinks like a stone, it's possible that you're not eating enough fibrous foods or drinking enough water. The meaner your diet is on fibre and fluid, the longer your faeces will take to travel the large intestine and the drier they will be when they reach daylight. If nature doesn't call often enough, wastes tend to become dehydrated and compressed into concrete pellets which are increasingly difficult to pass. The constipated result can be piles, diverticulitis or more serious bowel problems.

What you should be aiming for are medium brown, well-defined and plentiful blobs that plop out without straining, break up when they hit the water and float (or sink slowly) but flush away with ease. If you can manage some with unkempt or fluffy edges rather than smooth ones, then so much the better. Floating, by the way, is fine but if they bob like corks and resist the flush, this could mean that you're not absorbing the fat in your diet. Called steatorrhea, this is a serious condition that needs an immediate visit to the doctor. You should also seek medical advice if you notice that your stools are black (and you're not taking iron supplements or eating liquorice or beetroot), if your poo resembles ground coffee or if there is any blood on the paper or in the pan.

What frequency?

The late Dr Dennis Burkitt, famous fibre prescriber and the man responsible for bringing roughage to international attention through his work linking dietary fibre and cancer, said that it didn't matter how often one went but how much one passed per visit. Thirty years on, the concept has changed a little. If your diet is right, 'the more one goes, the more one delivers' is probably nearer to the truth of the matter.

What colour?

The delectable doctor John Collee, medical columnist for the *Observer*, suggests that the variations on brown are so wide that a decorator's colour chart might be useful!

Examples:

- Some iron supplements, especially those constipating ferrous sulphate tablets that are often given out on prescription, will make waste products appear darker, sometimes almost black. Because this type of iron is poorly absorbed, much of it ends up in the faeces instead of in the bloodstream.

- Liquorice sweets could add black bits to your cast-offs.

- But black could also be the result of bleeding in the stomach.

- Beetroot and dark berries, especially blueberries, bring interesting purple variations, and vitamin B2 can provide a touch of orange or greenish designer detail to your waste products (including your urine); both are harmless; indeed, they're beneficial.

- A yellow/green hue could be indicative of yesterday's curry but might also signal liver or gall-bladder problems, infectious diarrhoea or the side-effects of antibiotics.

- More seriously, tan, grey or porridge-coloured wastes can mean a blocked bile duct, problems of the pancreas or malabsorption of fats.

- Dark red usually points to bleeding in the large intestine and could be an early indication of colon cancer.

- Very bright red blood is more likely to be due to an anal fissure or haemorrhoid.

- Mucus or pus in the stools can indicate a number of conditions, including irritable bowel syndrome, diverticulitis, inflammation or abscess and, again, can be associated with gastrointestinal cancer.

- The healthiest hue is believed to be a medium brown.

It is important to be aware of what you've eaten in the past few days so you don't frighten yourself unnecessarily into a panic diagnosis. If you're unsure, ask the advice of your doctor or practice nurse.

Does your poo pooh?

Odour is also a guide to gut behaviour. In most cases, if yours pongs to the extent that no one else could possibly enter the lavatorial area until the extractor fan has run at full steam or all the windows are opened wide for several hours, then this could be an indication that all is not well in waste land. If faeces stays too long in the colon, it putrefies (goes off), creating just the right conditions for not-so-friendly bacteria to thrive. The little horrors have a delicious time feeding on your undigested left-overs, multiplying like crazy and swamping and destroying the friendly flora by spitting out loads of toxins.

As the build-up of toxicity reaches overload, the toxic waste seeps through the gut wall back into the bloodstream, just like industrial waste trickles undetected into water courses. The ecology of the river or stream is destroyed but no one notices anything is wrong until the fish begin to die or wildlife starts to produce tumours. The damaging effects of toxicity in the large colon are similarly underhand and can be just as dangerous.

Quite a lot of faecal matter sticks so fast to the gut wall that it is un-likely ever to move again. The remaining wastes that sludge and creak their way to the outside world are usually very concentrated, loaded with bacteria and, consequently, extremely smelly.

If you've read that God put the smell in farts for those who are hard of hearing, it isn't true. You might be surprised to learn that bodily wastes are not, naturally, unpleasant. Sure, they have their own particular odour, but if the diet is consistently healthy and there is the right balance of good bacteria in the gut, then any smell produced during farting or defaecating should neither linger for long nor require emergency fumigation!

An interesting act?

Frenchman Joseph Pujol (1857–1945) was an extraordinary music hall act who, at the height of his fame, was earning more at the box office than Sarah Bernhardt. His speciality was inhaling air through his anus and then, by controlling his abdominal and rectal muscles, farting recognisable tunes in different styles from violin to trombone. It's reported that his audiences, which often included royalty, were convulsed with laughter. It is also re-ported that his emissions were completely odourless.

Diet has a direct bearing on faecal odour. Although a vegetarian diet – because of its high-fibre content – can create a bit of flatus, a low-fibre diet or one high in meat can be disagreeably smelly as well as gassy. Researchers who compared the faeces of vegetarians to those of meat-eaters report that eliminations from omnivores (those whose diets include meat as well as vegetables) are far more potent than those from vegetarians. The reason is that animal products putrefy more readily than plant foods and, on their journey through the colon, produce the toxic gases that I described above. If your diet is high in fat, high in meat and/or low in fibre, your chances of stinky stools are much greater than if you have a low-fat, no-meat, high-fibre diet. Statistics also show that where meat consumption is high and fibre intake is low, colon cancer is high. In countries where the population consumes high levels of fibre but smaller quantities of meat, there is correspondingly less bowel disease.

VERY IMPORTANT POINT

Although bleeding is a common occurrence in bowel disorders and may not necessarily be a sign of serious disease, it is always wise to ask for a medical examination if you spot any. I make no apologies for repeating this: if you notice any bleeding, change of colour, swelling, stools that won't flush away or any change in bowel habit that concerns you, then please seek medical advice without delay. Never be embarrassed about discussing such matters with your GP. He or she will have seen more back-sides than you've had hot dinners. It's their job. Doctors would always rather you 'bothered' them unnecessarily than waited until it's too late for them to help you. A few seconds of awkwardness could, literally, save your life. And good news is great stuff – it puts your mind at rest.

Did you know?

The first water closet (WC) was invented by Sir John Harrington, godson to Queen Elizabeth 1, and installed at Kelston, near Bath in 1589. The invention of the modern flush loo is generally credited to two gentlemen – although lots of others had a hand in it. The first was Joseph Bramah in

1778, who must have done a good job; his name gave rise to the phrase 'a real Bramah'. The second fellow was Thomas Crapper who added his modifications in the 1860s. If you've connected his name with any modern vernacular, you'd be right! Working closely with another Thomas – Twyford (still famous today for bathroom furniture and fittings) – he produced the 'pull and go' cistern and brought toilets out into the open (out of elaborately engraved wooden surrounds, that is) to become the familiar pedestal design we know today. Quite an achievement in the Victorian age of prudery where piano legs were covered so as not to give offence!

I thought you might be wondering!

4.

How Long Does it Take?

❝ I have finally kum to the konklusion that a good reliable sett ov bowels is wurth more tu a man than enny [kwontity] ov brains. ❞

from *Josh Billings – His Sayings*, 1866 Henry Wheeler Shaw, 1818–1885

The movement of food from one end of the body to the other will vary enormously from person to person, depending upon the health and efficiency of his or her digestion and the type of food eaten. The whole thing is, quite literally, a moveable feast. However, because a healthy digestion and efficient, fast turnover are so important, it's worth repeating here that the longer the transit time, the greater the risk of a number of bowel diseases including constipation, diverticulosis and cancer of the colon.

Let's say you begin eating a meal at around 1 p.m. This is where you can be the most help to your overworked digestion, by chewing everything really thoroughly. Remember the old saying 'well chewed is already half digested'? My favourite way of describing this is to 'chew your liquids and drink your solids'. Sounds weird but give it some thought. If you *chew* your liquids, you move them around your mouth quite a few times before you swallow them. If you *drink* your solids, that means you've chewed them so well, they're practically liquid before you swallow them. Either way, whatever you put into your mouth has been well mixed with saliva (and those all important, starch-splitting enzymes).

I'd like to tell you here about a chap named Horace Fletcher (1849–1919) who was an early advocate of something he called 'industrious munching'. The story goes that Horace was refused life insurance because of his obesity but was eventually accepted after losing more than 18 kilos (40 pounds). His method? Chewing everything not just a few times but until it was smashed up into a semi-liquid and slipped down his gullet of its own accord. His theories were so popular that 'munching parties' were held and the chewing of each mouthful was timed with a stopwatch! I'm really not joking.

Take your time over a plate of food. If you've dealt with it in less than ten minutes, you're eating far too quickly. Fifteen to twenty minutes would be much more desirable.

Travelling time from the mouth to the stomach takes anything from three to ten seconds. When food arrives in the stomach, it's likely to stay there from forty-five minutes to several hours, depending upon the type of food you have eaten. Liquids travel through the fastest. Fruits are next. Vegetables take a bit longer than that. Starchy foods (carbohydrates) could stick around for a couple of hours. Proteins need to hang in there for a good four hours. This is only a guide, of course, and would apply only if every food or drink was taken separately. If different types of food are all chewed up and swallowed together, well, transit time is anyone's guess.

To work properly, the stomach needs to be relaxed, not under stress. That's why it helps if you sit down to eat and if you stay sitting down for at least ten minutes after you've finished. If you eat a reasonably sized meal in the middle of the day, you'd probably expect a healthy digestion to have dealt with the stomach stuff by around 5 p.m.

Once the food is in the small intestine, sorting and absorbing can take anything from two to four hours. But let's go with three hours for this meal. By my reckoning, the wastes should shuffle off into the large intestine at around 8 p.m.

Once through the ileo-caecal valve at the bottom of the small intestine, leftovers can take anything from five hours to several days to travel the last section of the journey through the large intestine or large colon. Here, waste liquids are converted into faeces. Most important of all, billions of bacteria manufacture B vitamins and vitamin K, as well as (I know you'll be surprised to hear this) lots of different gases! Bacteria also feed on undigested fibrous matter, reducing the quantity of faeces produced. The wastes that you pass are usually made up of about one-third bacteria.

In an ideal world, a meal should really take no longer than twelve hours to produce results! Two bowel movements in every twenty-four hours is about right in a healthy person. This doesn't necessarily mean that going only once a day is a really bad move, but speeding things up a little can only be good for your long-term health.

Page 80 has the low-down on what happens when a transit time of twelve hours extends to several days!

5.

Where Does it Hurt?

❛ A drug is a substance which, when injected into a rat, will produce a scientific report. ❜

Anon

Don't be nervous about a consultation or physical examination. The doctor will, truly, have lost count of the number of chests, abdomens and backsides he or she has examined. It's all in a day's work for them, so relax. A simple check-up could be all that is needed to put your mind at rest.

Communicating with your doctor

Ask your doctor or specialist to explain any examination or test before it happens. And do ask questions. We often come away from a consultation wondering what it was all about and wishing we'd mentioned this or asked about that.

It can be difficult not to feel nervous, afraid or intimidated but re-member that your medical advisers are there to help you. Some may be abrupt, others may seem preoccupied and everyone is always busy. All that can be hard to cope with when you're not feeling well, but it doesn't mean they don't have your best interests at heart. Describe your symp-toms using whichever words feel most comfortable to you, but be specific. The doctor won't expect you to use medical terminology. Tell them if you find nudity or physical examinations upsetting, if you're frightened or embarrassed or don't know what to say. They will really appreciate knowing you're struggling to describe your problem. If your religion or culture demands that you observe specific rituals when it comes to cleansing the body after examination or treatment, or during a stay in hospital, then tell the doctor or the nurse in charge.

It's comforting to know that most abdominal and chest pain is what doctors call 'self-limiting' – in other words, it will go away without the need for any treatment. However, if pain hits you hard and suddenly, or if you are suffering severe discomfort that has persisted for more than four hours, you should contact your doctor or local casualty department at once. If you're experiencing any kind of pain during pregnancy or if you have chest or abdominal pain that frightens or worries you, consider yourself an emergency and contact your local hospital emergency department or telephone the duty doctor without delay. **Any chest pain should be taken seriously** as it could be angina or the early signs of a heart attack – **especially if it is accompanied by pain in the arms**.

There may be nothing seriously wrong, but the distress caused, for example, by bloating or trapped wind can be excruciating and deceiving. Not only does the discomfort move around, but it can also be an amazing mimic. Get ghastly gas and you could imagine gallstones, appendicitis and a heart attack all within the space of an hour or two. It's always best to get yourself checked out.

Don't be afraid to go back. If you have persistent symptoms of any kind and a medical examination cannot find anything wrong, don't be afraid to bother the doctor again or ask for a second opinion. Quite recently, I met someone who, a few weeks earlier, had landed himself in hospital after collapsing in the street with a perforated ulcer and severe anaemia from internal bleeding – and this despite several surgery visits in preceding weeks complaining of tiredness and chest and stomach pain. So never be afraid to ask and ask again if you are not feeling any better. As a GP friend of mine says, doctors are not there to nag you or make you afraid, they are there to provide a service and the best of their medical knowledge.

Try complementary treatments

Get the best of both worlds. I believe wholeheartedly in a healing approach that utilises all that is best in both orthodox and complementary treatments. Although I still find myself concerned in equal measure about doctors who don't believe in alternative therapies, as well as about alternative therapists who think all orthodox treatments are bad or dangerous, it's extremely encouraging that so many GPs are now happy to refer patients to non-medical but, nonetheless, highly trained practitioners of holistic medicine, and also to welcome these treatments into the surgery setting.

In the not too distant past, therapies such as chiropractic, osteopathy, acupuncture, herbalism, homoeopathy, naturopathy and nutrition were being dismissed as quackery. As time went on, they were 'upgraded' to *fringe* medicine, until grudging acceptance that they might know what they were talking about eventually promoted them to *alternative*. Now that holistic and natural approaches have achieved such an enviable – and no longer dismissable – track record in restoring good health, conventional medicine has had no choice but to accept them as *complementary* to the mainstream.

Despite this progress, complaints of quackery still abound, usually, as you might have noticed, from medical men and women who don't understand or have no knowledge of the subject they are criticising. I think that most of this is born out of fear of losing control and perhaps status; but then that's just my opinion. I hear many, many horror stories about specialists who are scornful, pompous or aggressive. Their disease is called 'closed mind syndrome', its major symptom being arrogance. In the world of the know-it-all consultant, patients are an irritation or idiots who, despite the fact that they live every day in their own bodies, have no opinion of any value about their own illnesses.

Thankfully, there are other doctors with open minds. A specialist I saw just this month about my accident-damaged knees and spine was full of praise for natural treatments and recommended that I continue to take glucosamine sulphate and chondroitin sulphate. They're just as good as, if not better than, anti-arthritis drugs, and without side-effects, he tells me. He also prescribed acupuncture.

My own GP is tops on my list because he listens, keeps an open mind, respects the patient's opinion and feelings, and has a cracking sense of humour. But then I do think patients reap what they sow. If you approach your GP with a sour face, head hung down, asking no questions, never smiling and never asking the doctor how they are today, then it's much more difficult for them to feel a responsive empathy towards you, however hard they may be trying.

We're quick to complain when things go wrong but I wonder if, sometimes, our efforts to communicate with the doctor are just as inadequate as the doctor's efforts to communicate with us. I repeat my assertion that it is so important to work *with* your doctor. If you're currently on some kind of prescribed medication, for example, but want to try some of the alternatives that you've read or heard about, it's clearly not sensible to discontinue your prescription without discussing the situation and asking for his or her opinion and support. It's also important to accept the fact that, because they're unlikely to have had any training or experience in the natural approaches to a particular disease, you may need, actually, to educate your doctor. The Internet and libraries will always be excellent sources of scientific papers and medical and nutritional research. There are literally thousands of journals containing thousands of reports on successful studies using natural medicine. It's simply that doctors don't get to hear about them, mostly due to lack of time to locate them, and because their only major source of information comes from pharmaceutical company literature and 'drug reps' who visit them in the surgery.

Go surfing and researching and obtain copies of reports concerning the treatment that interests you, then show them to your doctor. In the event that your efforts are ignored, you might have to consider changing to another GP or another practice. Don't be browbeaten or intimidated.

When we first moved to the area we are currently living in and I needed to sign on with a new doctor, I went searching and dismissed three before finding my present GP. One was pleasant enough but completely opposed to alternative ideas. The second explained that he couldn't do house calls in my area (who wants a doctor who won't come out in an emergency?). And I never did get to see the third one because, when I explained to the receptionist that I just wanted to meet the doctor before deciding whether or not to sign on (a recommendation made by my previous GP), she wouldn't allow me even the briefest of appointments unless I had something wrong with me.

At the first consultation with my new doctor, I explained that I had a particular interest in natural medicine and wanted to know if, following discussion, he would support me in my treatment choices. The answer was yes. I also told him I was only interested in signing on with a doctor who had a sense of humour and asked if he had one. Yes, he said, except on Mondays. It was, of course, a Monday. We laughed. I knew I'd found the right place.

6.

What's Up?
Acid Reflux

❝ [The effect of] gastric acid . . . [on] the lining of the oesophagus is like taking a bath in the drainings of automobile batteries. ❞

The Second Brain, Michael D. Gershon, MD, 1999

Read this chapter if you think you suffer from indigestion or think you might have acid reflux or the following:

- Dyspepsia
- Gastritis
- Heartburn
- Hiatus hernia
- Gastro-oesophageal reflux disease (GORD)
- Peptic ulcer

The number of different names used to describe digestive discomfort can be confusing. You know the sort of thing we usually associate with burning pain in the stomach or chest or gullet? Perhaps you think of it as heartburn. Someone else may say 'indigestion'. Doctors usually describe it as dyspepsia. Whatever we call it, we're probably trying to describe the uncomfortable results of a meal that disagreed with us. Maybe they were due to self-inflicted overindulgence. We'll groan and moan and we'll probably do it again, but heck, we enjoyed it, and anyway, occasional dietary stupity isn't life-threatening. In most cases, staying off the rich stuff and resting the digestion is all that is needed. But there are occasions when that dyspepsia can be a sign of a digestive system under strain, and that requires investigation and treatment.

Common signs and symptoms of poor digestion are given below. Those in bold type tend to be associated specifically with low levels of stomach acid (see page 39), as well as with other aspects of poor digestion and absorption.

Acne
Belching/flatulence
Bloating
Broken capillaries on the cheeks and the nose
Burning sensation in the chest
Constant fatigue
Dark circles under the eyes
Disturbed gut flora
Erratic bowel movements
Intestinal parasites
Nausea after meals, and especially after taking supplements
Rectal itching
Recurring anaemia
Sense of fullness after meals
Sensitivity to certain foods
Undigested matter in faeces
Weak, split, ridged or peeling fingernails
Yeast overgrowth/thrush

Jargon buster

Dyspepsia isn't a specific condition but is symptomatic of a number of different diseases. It's actually defined as 'any symptom of, disorder of or abuse of the digestive system that results in burning pain or discomfort in the upper abdomen, chest or gullet, with or without nausea, bloating, flatulence or burping'. Discomfort may be mild and infrequent, intermittent, or intense and constant. Symptoms can be the result of a stomach ulcer, or can occur where there is no evidence of ulceration – called non-ulcer dyspepsia. Varying degrees of dyspepsia may also be linked to gallstones, gastritis, gastro-oesophageal reflux disease (GORD), hiatus hernia, irritable bowel syndrome or diabetes, as well as the side-effects of some drugs and, more seriously, stomach cancer and disorders of the pancreas. Or they may just be the result of a terrible diet of rich, rushed, fatty, sugary foods. The pain of angina is often mistaken for dyspepsia which is why, of course, it's also called heartburn.

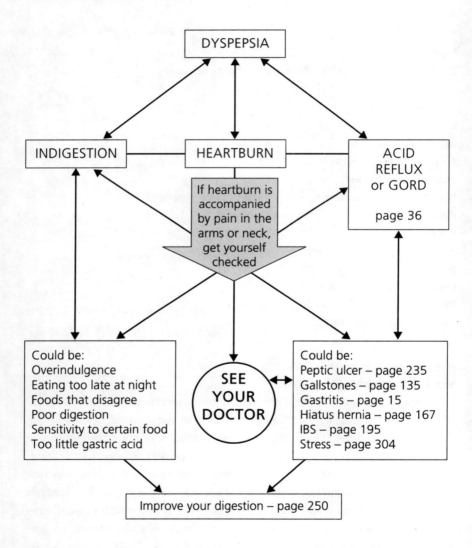

Because there are so many possible reasons for dyspepsia, tracking down the trigger usually requires a bit of detective work. That's why, just in case there's something serious going on, I always say to alert your doctor if:

- You find you need to use antacid medicines every day or after every meal.

- You regurgitate acid every day or every night.

- Pain wakes you during the night.

- You have any kind of pain brought on by physical activity.

- You have have unexplained shortness of breath, dizziness or nausea.

- The pain radiates from your chest into your neck and arms – or from the centre to the lower right side of your abdomen.

- There is loss of appetite or difficulty swallowing.

- There is any sudden or unexpected weight loss.

- You notice red blood or anything that resembles coffee grounds in your stools.

- Any of your symptoms are unrelenting and recurring.

This all sounds very alarmist, doesn't it? But I should emphasise that having dyspepsia doesn't necessarily indicate the presence of serious disease. It's simply that early diagnosis allows for the best chance of good and complete recovery. And – whatever you may think – doctors always prefer you to bother them unnecessarily than not make an appointment in the first place.

Perhaps there isn't *enough* acid?

It's not unusual for people suffering from acid reflux to actually have *low* levels of hydrochloric acid. The condition is easy to misdiagnose because so many of the symptoms are similar to those of over-acidity. The production of stomach juices tends to decrease as we age and is believed to be common in those over sixty.

Hypochlorhydria = reduced levels of hydrochloric acid.
Achlorhydria = no hydrochloric acid at all.

Signs of there being not enough hydrochloric acid can include:

Anal irritation
Bad breath
Bloating
Burning discomfort (called pyrosis)
Constipation
Flatulence
Foul-smelling farts
Metallic taste in the mouth
Nausea
Peeling or ridged nails
Sensitivity to certain foods
Skin problems, especially acne or red blotches on the cheeks or nose
Sore tongue
Symptoms associated with candidiasis, parasites and disturbed gut flora
Undigested food in the stools
Upper chest pain

Based on these signs, a visit to the doctor could easily result in a prescription for unnecessary antacids. So if your present medication is not helping you, talk again to your GP. There are simple tests available to practitioners that can determine whether you are producing too much or too little hydrochloric acid. If it's found that you're producing too little, supplements of hydrochloric acid can be taken with meals. However, don't even think about trying this unless you have talked to your doctor or nutritional adviser and undergone the necessary tests.

Too much acid?

Some people are unlucky enough to suffer from severe acidity. If this happens almost every day or after every meal, or if symptoms are persistent and involve frequent regurgitation of acid, doctors usually call the condition gastro-oesophageal reflux disease, or GORD. Unfortunately, every time I hear this silly acronym, I cannot help but think of the vegetable gourd.

Acid reflux occurs when the lower oesophageal sphinctre (the LES) doesn't close properly and allows the stomach's acidic contents to flow back, or 'reflux', into the defenceless gullet. This isn't supposed to happen, of course. Think back to page 14 where I explained that this doorway at the bottom of the lift shaft is designed to prevent the stomach contents from flowing upwards because it works like a one-way valve. It's closed most of the time and only opens momentarily as food arrives at the doorway and a nerve reflex 'turns the key'.

Jargon buster

Gastro-oesophageal reflux disease (GORD) is the latest medical jargon for acid reflux, and is sometimes used as an alternative term for heartburn. In countries where oesophagus is spelt differently (as esophagus), the letters change slightly to GERD. Another term that means the same thing is reflux oesophagitis; that is, reflux into the oesophagus causing an 'itis' = inflammation. For simplicity, I've used the more familiar terms, acid reflux and GORD, throughout the relevant sections of this book.

Who is at risk?

Anyone can get GORD, or acid reflux. But these groups tend to be most at risk:

- Pregnant mums.

- The overweight.

- Smokers.

- Babies – because little ones don't have a fully developed oesophageal sphinctre. Their tendency to bring back their food usually lessens in the first few months of life as the digestive system matures and the muscles get stronger.

- Sufferers of hiatus hernia, gallstones, gastritis or constipation.

- Anyone who has poor-quality digestion.

Did you know?

The burning sensation that we know as heartburn is so-called because it occurs in the upper chest. It's the same thing as acid reflux and is also sometimes called dyspepsia, but it actually has nothing whatsoever to do with the heart; it's caused by stomach juices, mixed with semi-liquid food, pushing past the doorway between the stomach and the oesophageal sphinctre and burning the unprotected gullet.

What aggravates acid reflux?

- The tendency to reflux is exacerbated if the stomach is overfull, if acids are produced in excess or at the wrong time, or when there is increased pressure in or on the stomach. However, this will only occur if our friend LES is already slack or if there is a hiatus hernia.

- Gravity can also pay a part if the doorway is open even a crack and we happen to be bending forwards or lying down at the time. A tiny amount of reflux may cause no problem because the area just above the sphincter contains glands that will secrete enough alkaline juices to neutralise the acid. And in any event, the oesophagus has an amazing ability for self-repair. But repeated attacks or larger quantities of acid will cause pain and burning and, eventually, erosion of the unprotected lining of the gullet.

- Eating a large meal late at night or lying down too soon after eating can also result in a sore gullet and, in some cases, a sore throat. If this happens often enough, the acid will damage the lining of the gullet. As we saw during our journey through the digestive system (see page 10), the stomach lining is designed to withstand the strong action of hydrochloric acid which it produces to help break down food substances; the gullet, however, isn't so well protected.

Bornholm disease

The discomfort associated with a condition known as Bornholm disease can be mistaken for oesophagitis or even for a heart attack. It is, however, completely unrelated, being a virus that causes sore throat, inflammation and spasms of pain in the neck, chest or upper abdomen.

Barrett's oesophagus

Barrett's oesophagus, discovered by British surgeon N.R. Barrett in 1950, is also relatively rare, affecting less than 5 per cent of people with hiatus hernia. I mention it here because the two main symptoms are acid reflux and regurgitation of food. The gullet is attacked repeatedly by stomach acid and pepsin. And even when there is no food in the stomach, sufferers can experience bitter reflux into the throat and mouth. If left untreated, this can progress to dysphagia (difficulty in swallowing), together with penetrating pain in the chest and between the shoulder blades. This usually indicates scarring or ulceration of the oesophagus. Treatment is nearly always essential and urgent in order to prevent internal bleeding and perforation of the ulcer into the chest cavity and lungs.

Experts are still unsure as to the causes of Barrett's oesophagus. What they do know is that, instead of the tough, acid-resistant lining at the very lower end of the gullet, just where it joins the stomach, the cells are much more like those of the stomach, susceptible to acid attack but without the protective mucous membrane. Because of the seriousness of this condition, it is advisable for patients with severe acid reflux or persistent hiatus hernia symptoms to undergo extensive tests if for no other reason than to rule out Barrett's oesophagus.

Likely symptoms of acid reflux

- A burning pain in the chest which most of us would describe as heartburn. If you've ever experienced that 'have-to-sit-up' sensation during the night, the chances are that some acid has squirted up into your gullet.

- A sour taste in the mouth – the result of acid returning as far as the pharynx (throat).

- Repeating or burping.

- Hoarseness of the voice, and because acid reflux can irritate the larynx (the voice box), some sufferers complain that it seems harder to breathe.

See your doctor

Acid reflux can be treated in several ways. Many people respond extremely well to dietary and lifestyle changes. For others, medication – and in rare situations, surgery – are options. You may already be under the care of your doctor for acid reflux. However, if you've been suffering from any of the symptoms detailed here for longer than a week or so and things haven't improved, don't hesitate to make an appointment with your health centre or surgery.

If you're not making progress with existing treatment, discuss this with your doctor. If you have not responded to medication or if symptoms are severe, further tests may include an endoscopy, which is usually carried out at a hospital day centre. This is a painless procedure that involves swallowing a thin, flexible tube, allowing a doctor to have a really good look around your gullet, stomach and the first section of your small intestine. You will be given a light sedative before the test and may need to spend a few hours resting afterwards. Make sure that someone goes with you to the hospital and takes you home again as you won't be allowed to drive on that day. It's likely that you could also be tested for *Helicobacter pylori*, the bacteria now known to be responsible for the majority of ulcers. This can be done using a simple breath test or blood test.

What medicines are available?

Antacids

You'll probably be given antacids in the form of aluminium hydroxide, magnesium salts, calcium carbonate or sodium bicarbonate. These simple alkalis are the most familiar drugs prescribed for acid reflux. They work by neutralising the acid but because the effect is short-lived and the symptoms often return when you stop using them, you may find that you need to take them after every meal. Different products vary in their action so if one doesn't work, it's always worth considering another. Side-effects include flatulence and changes in bowel habit. Antacids that contain magnesium can cause diarrhoea; those that contain aluminium may leave you constipated.

Protective drugs

You might be offered protective drugs in the form of tablets or liquids that coat the oesophagus and stomach lining, helping to prevent that acid attack. Most of these are based on alginates (made from seaweed), but they may also contain aluminium hydroxide and bicarbonates. Like the antacids above, they deal only with the symptoms, which may return once the medicine has been washed away.

Antispasmodics

Antispasmodics, which are often peppermint-based, treat the acid reflux by reducing the tension – or spasm – in the stomach wall. They can also help to reduce the feeling of fullness. Side-effects are few although, un-fortunately, peppermint can aggravate reflux in some people. If you are one of them, don't be afraid to mention this to your doctor.

Drugs to reduce acid secretion

If the more simple medicines don't make any difference, those that re-duce acid secretion are usually the next option. Scientific research tells us that a powerful natural chemical substance called histamine stimulates the release of gastric juices. Drugs called H2 receptor-antagonists, such as cimetidine or ranitidine, block the action of histamine and so help to re-duce both the quantity and the acidity of stomach acid. This family of drugs is usually well tolerated, although side-effects including headaches, dizziness, dry mouth, skin rashes, constipation, diarrhoea and fatigue can occur. There may also be a reduction in the absorption of some nutrients. Long-term use is definitely not recommended and ulcers may return when the medication is discontinued. This family of drugs may not be recommended if you are already taking certain types of asthma medica-tion or blood-thinning drugs.

Proton pump inhibitors

A stronger family of drugs known as proton pump inhibitors – omepra-zole, lansoprazole and pantoprazole – acts on the enzyme that triggers acid secretion and stops acid being produced altogether. Side-effects may include nausea, constipation, diarrhoea, gas, headaches, dizziness and skin rashes. Inevitably, without the presence of stomach acid to help in the breakdown of food, proteins will not be properly digested, and absorption of nutrients will be affected. Any drug that blocks the production of any substance that is usually considered essential to natural functioning, even if that drug effectively removes the symptoms, should be carefully monitored and never considered suitable for long-term use.

Antibiotics

Where the *Helicobacter pylori* are confirmed, a course of antibiotics, usually together with acid-suppressing medication, is the most likely prescription. Once the bacteria have been eradicated it's likely that the ulcer will heal and the need for further drugs will become unnecessary.

Both the H_2 receptor-antagonists and proton pump inhibitors have, for a long time, been the treatment of choice for ulcers, and they are indeed effective at healing peptic ulceration – but unless antibiotics are prescribed simultaneously to eradicate the *H. pylori* bacteria, H_2 antagonists may have limited success.

As a direct result of hearing about the experiences of so many patients who have been given repeat anti-ulcer drug prescriptions without regular consultation or check-up, I would like to reiterate the following concerns. Short-term treatment using one or more of these medicines can provide excellent results, but extended use is not advisable. If you've been taking your prescription for more than three months without seeing your doctor, make an appointment and have another chat. Acid-suppressing medication, if used extensively or unwisely, can mask symptoms rather than cure disease. The best chance of avoiding a recurrence of acid reflux problems is to combine medical advice with sensible changes to lifestyle and diet that ultimately heal the existing problem and prevent repetition.

Note that some of the medicines discussed in this chapter are available over the counter without prescription. Others are prescription-only. If you have any questions about any of them, talk to a pharmacist or your doctor.

For more information on the treatment of ulcers see page 235.

Action plan for acid reflux

Your diet

Here are some tips on specific improvements that you can make to your diet.

Don't overdo the dairy

It's one of those odd dietary ironies that the foods you think might be the most helpful can be those that give the least relief – and vice versa. Although now out-dated, an oft-prescribed 'antacid' was milk, recommended by many a medic in years past for ulcerated stomachs and sore gullets. Now we know that cow's milk can actually increase the production of stomach acid, so if you suffer from acid reflux, milk really is best avoided. For some people, however, giving up all cow's milk products makes the biggest and best difference to their symptoms. Others may find that yoghurts and cheeses, especially those made from sheep's or goat's milk, cause no problems. The only way to find out is to experiment.

Get fresh with a new diet

Fruits and vegetables were, until not all that long ago, a no-no for ulcers because it was believed they aggravated acid production. But the acid in the fruits we eat is not the same as the acid in our stomachs. To suggest otherwise is to completely misunderstand the process of digestion. Although some 'sharp' fruits such as citrus, plums and rhubarb are not well digested by some sensitive stomachs, it's now accepted that an increased intake of fresh produce can do more to correct acid production than the once-favoured bland diet. Promise yourself you'll eat at least five servings a day of fresh fruits, vegetables and salad foods. It sounds a lot but it isn't much. These foods are rich in fibre and packed with nutrients. They're usually much more efficiently digested than high-fat snacks and heavy-duty protein foods like meat. *But . . .*

Avoid citrus fruits for a while

The most troublesome of all the foods is, in my experience, packaged orange juice. This again has nothing to do with stomach acid but is due to the fact that orange juice is a common allergen that is not well digested. So before you go mad and give up lemons, grapefruits and limes as well, just try easing up on the orange juice first. If you are very sensitive to citric acid and other acidic foods, you might find it helpful to avoid vinegar, salad dressings and anything containing citric acid (E330 on food labels) until symptoms ease. By the way, cooked and canned tomatoes tend to be more acid-producing than raw, skinned salad tomatoes.

Take some Molkosan

This lactic acid whey can help to regulate both overacidity and underacidity. Take a teaspoon of Molkosan in a glass of water or juice just before meals. It is available from health food stores. See my notes on whey on page 302. For stockist information, see Bioforce in the Resource section (page 323).

Try food combining

Sometimes it isn't a single ingredient in the diet that causes acid but the combination of foods. For example, one of the worst perpetrators of stomach discomfort can be indigestible mixtures such as acid fruits mixed with starchy foods (fruit pies). Thinking carefully about how you plan your meals and how you combine them may be all that is necessary to bring about an improvement. Food combining is a simple system that involves not mixing proteins and starches at the same meal. Feedback from readers of my food-combining books and from former patients suggests very strongly indeed that this type of healthy diet improves the way the body digests its food, thereby reducing acid production, improving stomach emptying, speeding transit time and helping to achieve a balanced body weight.

For more information on food combining see page 283.

Cut back on fat

A high-fat diet is likely to aggravate acid reflux because fats take a long time to digest, delaying stomach emptying and often calling up excess quantities of stomach juices. Try to avoid high-fat foods, especially take-away 'fast' foods such as burgers, chips, pies and pizzas loaded with cheese.

Grill rather than fry

Throw away that frying pan and/or deep-fat fryer. Go for grilling or stir-frying instead.

Take a break between bites

Remember our journey through the digestive system (see page 10)? The faster you eat, the harder your stomach has to work and the more likely you are to suffer from heartburn. Empty you mouth completely and wait a moment or two before you start on the next bite.

Give some thought to planning your meals

This will ensure you don't find yourself with an empty refrigerator, or rushing to grab a bite between between appointments. It's at times like these that fast foods and junk snacks are a big temptation.

Beware
These foods may be best avoided or kept to a minimum if you have acid reflux

Alcohol	Cow's milk	Onions	Rhubarb
Caffeine	Fatty foods	Peppermint	Salad dressings
Chillis	Fruit pies	Peppers	Spices
Citrus fruits and juices	Garlic	Plums	Tomatoes

Go for it !
Check out *If You Do Nothing Else . . .* starting on page 250 for more tips on what's good for a healthy digestion and what's best avoided.

Take care not to restrict your diet

The foods listed in the box opposite are those that are most often reported by sufferers to cause problems. But everyone is an individual and what applies to one person may not apply to another. So please don't think that you need to remove them all from your diet. You could be restricting a particularly nutritious food for no good reason. If you suspect that a particular food may be causing you grief, exclude it for a couple of weeks and reintroduce it before you assess any improvements. Then only leave it out completely if you're sure it's a real trigger.

Don't spice up your life

Hot spices and peppery foods can aggravate acid in some people. Packaged foods, especially ready-made meals and prepacked soups, are often very high in pepper, salt and other strong flavourings. If your digestion is under pressure, skip the spices for a while – and that goes for whether you're eating out or eating in. 'Cooler' spices such as coriander, cumin and cardamom may still suit you. The only way to find out is to experiment.

Cut out the caffeine

It's seriously bad news for heartburn sufferers. Learn to drink less tea and coffee and opt for soda drinks that don't contain caffeine. Try lots of different kinds of herbal and fruit teas; add grated fresh root ginger and a little Manuka honey to them. Delicious! And drink more water.

Don't hit the bottle or the six-pack

Excess alcohol can aggravate a number of different digestive and bowel disorders and is very likely to bring on attacks of acid reflux. Beer and spirits may increase symptoms more severely than wine so I would suggest that you stick to a max of one glass of wine a day or give up entirely to see if symptoms go away.

What else can you do?

There are other things apart from dietary improvements that you should do if you suffer from heartburn or acid reflux.

Pack it in, give it up, quit

If you smoke, do whatever it takes to stop. Tell yourself you'll do it right now, for the sake of your health – or because you're fed up with smelling like an old ashtray, because it isn't good for the people around you, because it's bad for your health in general, because it wreaks havoc on your digestion and because you want to live a longer, healthier life. Who needs a reason! Tobacco chemicals cause us to over-produce stomach acid (too much acid is as bad as too little), reducing the rate at which the stomach empties and preventing the oesophageal sphincter from working properly. If you're a smoker with heartburn, I'm sure you'll have worked it out for yourself that cigarettes worsen the symptoms.

Lose a little weight

If you're carrying more kilos than you should be, shedding them will do your digestion a big favour. That's because spare tyres around the abdominal cavity increase the pressure inside it and continually push the stomach contents (and, of course, the acid) upwards into the gullet.

Give your gut some space

Relax that waistband. Loosen that belt. Forget the tight jeans or the grippy girdle. Constricting clothing literally squeezes the body inwards, pushes the stomach contents upwards and increases the risk of acid reflux.

Take time out

Constant stress can affect your digestive processes and cause higher levels of stomach acid to be produced, even when there is no food in your stomach. Learn to relax and to look after yourself.

Did you know?
A unit is half a pint of beer, one glass of wine or one tot of spirits. And, by the way, avoiding alcohol all week only to binge on seven units during a weekend is definitely not recommended for anyone, whether you suffer from heartburn or not.

For more information on stress see page 304.

Get moving

Together with a healthier diet, regular activity could help to take the pressure off your abdomen and improve digestive function by trimming fat and toning muscle. Half an hour a day, walking briskly around the block or across the park, could make a big difference. Walk, don't run. If you've just eaten a gentle stroll is fine, but leave an hour before taking strenuous exercise.

Don't be a pillpopper

Over-the-counter and prescription remedies can be very helpful at getting you through a bad attack of acid reflux. One of the best 'gut soothers' is bismuth-based Pepto-Bismol. In my experience it is gentle, produces rapid effects, and as far as I'm aware carries no serious side-effects. But no antacid should be considered more than a very occasional short-term option. If you're troubled regularly by any of the symptoms listed above, make an appointment to see your doctor and ask for a check-up or a second opinion. Repeated attacks of acid reflux are your body's way of telling you that something isn't right. It's better to get help and to change your diet and lifestyle than to live on antacid medication.

Try using natural antacids

Natural antacids can be just as effective as drug medicines, and there are a number of drug-free remedies available for the treatment of acidity. The plant remedy slippery elm can help to soothe a stroppy stomach. Try Blackmores or Bio-Health Slippery Elm. Bioforce Silicea – a tablespoon of gel in a glass of water taken fifteen minutes before eating – puts a protective lining over the digestive tract. I have also found that Biocare Gastroplex or Potters Acidosis, taken after meals, can be very effective. So too is Blackmores Celloid Mineral Sodium Phosphate, which helps to buffer excess acidity. If a deficiency of stomach acid is suspected, Blackmores Celloid Mineral Chloride Compound or Blackmores Digestive Aid helps to stimulate digestive juices. The Resource Directory on page 323 has stockist information.

Take care at night

For most sufferers, the symptoms of acid reflux can be worst while they are lying down asleep. Allowing the situation to go untreated disturbs your rest, and repeated attacks of reflux can lead to serious health problems, including bleeding or ulcers in the oesophagus. Acid can also regurgitate into the lungs, creating breathing difficulties and increasing the risk of infections. A small percentage of sufferers may also develop a more serious condition known as Barrett's oesophagus (see page 43). If you wake up sputtering, have an early morning sore throat or an acid taste in the mouth, or feel that your breathing is restricted in any way, don't delay seeing your GP.

Don't eat late

Try to get your evening meal done and dusted by 8 p.m. And don't eat crap food late – especially not burgers, chips, pizzas, salted snacks or chocolate. A light snack such as a yoghurt or some fruit an hour before you intend to sleep should be fine, but anything heavier is going to cause you hassle. If, for example, you eat a packet of crisps just before you go to bed they will not be digested before you get horizontal.

Look after your back

Spinal misalignment can be the cause of acid reflux. If your over-acidity is accompanied by back problems, a visit to the chiropractor or osteopath could be worth while. Also replace your pillow regularly. It can be worth paying extra for a firmer design that keeps its shape and supports your neck and spine in the correct position.

Reduce the risk of a night-time attack

If night-time attacks are a problem for you, try raising the head of your bed by around 10 centimetres (3–4 inches), but make sure that anything you use for this purpose is firm and not likely to give way. Placing an additional ordinary pillow immediately under your existing pillow is not

53

always a good idea because it tends to push your spine out of line during sleep and can result in neck stiffness or back pain. A better option may be to place an extra pillow between the mattress and the bed base. Alternatively, buy a purpose-made wedge that fits under the pillow end of your mattress.

Reducing the risk of acid reflux

KATHRYN'S TOP TEN TIPS

1. Eat smaller meals.

2. Quit smoking.

3. Chew food thoroughly.

4. Give up cow's milk.

5. Cut right back on coffee.

6. Try food combining.

7. Give up alcohol, at least for a while.

8. Don't eat fruits and carbohydrates at the same meal.

9. Reduce the fat in your diet.

10. If you're overweight, try losing a little of the excess weight.

WWW

Just as I was completing *Good Gut Healing*, I came across a really excellent little book called *Tell Me What To Eat If I Have Acid Reflux*, which I spotted quite by chance in a second-hand bookshop. It's an American title by Elaine Magee and is published by New Page Books. Since then, I've been onto the Internet and found that it's available from **www.amazon.co.uk.** Go to www.amazon.com if you're outside the United Kingdom or try the author's own website **www.recipedoctor.com.** The book includes excellent recipes which I think could be really helpful for anyone who suffers from acid reflux or any of the related conditions I've been talking about.

7.

What's Up?
Bloating and Gas

6 Okay. We'll take a couple of twink-dinks, four chocco-goos, a litre of belchacola, ten bags of deep-fried fat stix . . . then we're off to taunt the ol' digestive system. 9

Eating Alive – Prevention Thru Good Digestion, Dr Jonn Matsen, 1991

Read this chapter if you have bloating and gas, or suspect that you have any of these:

- Candida
- Irritable bowel syndrome
- Diverticulitis

When the abdomen feels full and distended, we call the condition 'bloating'. It's most often caused by a build-up of intestinal gas. If you burp it up, with or without the fine fragrance of your last meal, it's known as flatulence. If you expel it downwards, perhaps with an even cheaper scent, it's called flatus or, more familiarly, farting.

The good news is that all kinds of bloating usually respond really well to dietary changes. I hope that the advice in this chapter and in related sections will help you to reduce pain, pressure and the misery of a bloated abdomen.

Who is at risk?

Anyone at any age can suffer from it.

What aggravates it?

Incomplete digestion

Overeating

Lactose intolerance

Constipation

Disturbed balance of gut flora

Swallowing air (aerophagy)

Talking while chewing

Chewing gum

Inadequate chewing

Eating too quickly

Inadequate digestive enzymes

Poor liver function

Other health disorders associated with bloating

Candidiasis (yeast overgrowth)

Diverticular disease

Irritable bowel syndrome (IBS)

Bowel obstruction

Crohn's disease

Ulcerative colitis

Oedema (fluid retention)

Completely normal

Most of us, quite naturally, feel embarrassed if we suffer with mild or occasional gas but it really is the most normal occurrence and nothing to be ashamed of. Nor is it always a sign of ill health – it's simply a way of relieving internal pressure. According to Dr John Collee, most excellent medical columnist and now author and scriptwriter, 'thirteen farts or an average of half a litre of gas per day is quite normal and can be a pleasure'. Other experts suggest that between fifteen and twenty per day are nearer the mark.

Pleasures aside, whether or not flatulence, or flatus, can be considered 'normal' really depends on what you've eaten, how well you digest, how efficiently you eliminate and what it smells like! It's when the occasional mini-burp, king-size belch or sneaky fart becomes persistent and ongoing that it could be time to take action.

What's that smell?

Persistently odorous discharges are not only unpleasant for everyone else, but they may also not be such a healthy sign for you either, especially if the results of your visits clear the precincts or render the lavatory, washroom, bathroom, loo, toilet or outhouse impassable for several hours each day.

Come on now. No giggling. Take a deep breath and pull yourself together. Bloating is no laughing matter. Trapped air can create the most excruciating pressure and discomfort, so bad that it has sometimes been mistaken for many a more serious condition. It can feel as if it's caught up under the diaphragm, deep in the abdominal cavity or even beneath the collarbone. When it seems as if gas isn't actually in your digestive system at all but somewhere else entirely, the most likely explanation is that the pressure in the gut is causing pain to be radiated out to other areas.

Gas can get into your intestine in various ways:

- Chewing gum.

- Talking with your mouth full.

- Swallowing air when you're anxious.

- Opening up the abdomen during surgery can bring on agonising bouts of trapped post-operative gas.

- Carbohydrates (starchy, sugary foods) can produce gas in the large intestine through a process called fermentation. Fruit sugar, the main carbohydrate in fruits, can ferment in your large intestine, causing you to feel bloated. Fruits themselves are a common cause of intestinal gas, most often if they are eaten with certain other foods. In particular, starchy foods and fruits make an extremely gassy combination.

- Foods that aren't properly digested in the small intestine will be attacked by bacteria in the large intestine where leftovers ferment and produce gas as a by-product. The situation can be made worse if friendly gut flora – responsible for keeping the system sweet smelling – is in short supply. There is more on this on page 294.

- High-fibre diets, onions and, as everyone knows, beans are notorious sources of fiery flatus!

- Fatty foods can create gas if they aren't broken down properly in the small intestine.

- Failing to chew food properly can lead to inadequate digestion, which in turn encourages bacterial overgrowth and consequent gas.

> For more information on friendly flora see the section on probiotics, page 294.

The brewery in your bellly

If you binge on the 'chocco-goo' or overdo the sugar a windy bowel can produce alcohol just as efficiently as your favourite beer keller. The phenomenon is known as 'auto-brewery syndrome' (no, I'm really not kidding) and depends of the level, type and activity of bacteria and yeast organisms living in our guts.

Aerophagy

Nearly everyone swallows air when they eat. Some people swallow air even when they're not eating. It's called aerophagy. Watch those who eat too quickly or who talk with their mouths full, and their conversation is likely to be punctuated with the need to expel air.

Does milk upset you?

A common cause of bloating and gas is a condition known as lactose intolerance. This is the inability to properly digest the natural sugar (lactose) found in milk.

> For more information on lactose intolerance see page 215.

Action plan for bloating and gas

Improve your digestion

Take steps to improve the way your body digests its food, such as chewing every mouthful really thoroughly, sitting down to eat and not rushing around immediately after food. This may all sound boringly simple but these changes can make an amazing difference. The chapter If You Do Nothing Else . . . is essential reading (see page 250).

Check your posture

Sitting in a slumped or cramped position restricts your digestive organs and can trap the gas.

Chew with your mouth closed

Also don't talk when you're eating. An open mouth draws in air, increasing the risk of bloating and burping.

Give up the gum

If you suffer from bloating, flatulence or belching, manage without this notorious gas maker.

Can the cans

All that canned fizz isn't just full of sugar and loaded with additives, it's also pumped with bubbles. The very action of drinking from the can could make bloating and burping much worse.

Did you know?
A human of average size contains 40 litres (9 gallons) of water, enough carbon to make 9,000 pencil leads, enough phosphorous for 8,000 boxes of matches, enough iron for 5 nails, enough salt to fill 6 salt cellars and enough hydrogen to fill a balloon capable of lifting the body to the top of Mount Snowdon?

Take time over your meals

Gobbling your food means you'll probably gobble down loads of air, too.

Dentures? Make they fit properly

Shovelling your tongue around your mouth to check on your dentures is a common cause of air swallowing.

Don't boot the fruit

Avoiding fruit means that you're missing out on all those wonderful nutrients which are so important for your good health. But eating fruit with other food or after the main course can result in them not getting properly digested, and being left to ferment and produce gas. So it's not to be recommended. Instead of giving fruit up, try eating them in a different way. Like this:

- As a starter – at the very beginning of a meal when your stomach is actually empty. The fruits may have a better chance of getting away into the lower sections of the intestines and being digested before other food arrives in the stomach. This may appear unconventional but is a tip that seems to work if you're prepared to leave ten or fifteen minutes between any fruit starter and the main course. If you suffer from irritable bowel syndrome, see my notes about fruits on page 284.

- Chew all fruits really thoroughly. Although fruit peel can provide excellent dietary fibre, it may be best discarded.

- If you're suffering from any kind of digestive distress, such as bloating or acid reflux, don't mix fruit with raw vegetable or salad dishes. No one really knows why, but there is quite a lot of anecdotal evidence to suggest that this combination can increase the risk of flatulence and wind pain.

- As a snack, fruit with sheep's or goat's milk yoghurt is said by some sufferers to be an easily digestible combination.

- Whatever you do, avoid mixing fruit with starchy foods such as bread, rice or pastry.

Helpful hint

If you find that milk bloats you up (and this can happen even if you're not lactose intolerant) try substituting cow's milk yoghurt with sheep's or goat's milk yoghurt. Some people find sheep's and goat's milk products easier to digest than cow's milk products. It's been estimated that just one fluid ounce of undigested milk will produce around 50 millilitres (ten teaspoons) of gas in a normal intestine. Where the bad microbes are running riot and the good bacteria are in short supply, the amount expands a hundred times to an explosive 5,000 millilitres (that's well over 4 litres/1 gallon of gas!).

Beware
Foods that are known to cause bloating and gas
Milk
Cheese
Cow's milk yoghurt
Wheat bran
Sugar
Products made with wheat flour such as bread, biscuits,
    buns, pastry and cakes
Beans
Vegetables including broccoli, cauliflower, beetroot, onions
    and spinach
Some fruits
Chewing gum, both regular and sugar-free

Don't restrict your diet

Many of the foods listed in the box above are rich in a wide range of nutrients and as such can be an important part of a healthy diet. Imagine what would happen if you gave up all such foods completely. The chances are extremely high that you would become severely malnourished and at risk of far more than just bloating and gas. I've given you the list so that you can try to isolate which foods, if any, cause you most problems. But it isn't exclusive. It may be that you've already discovered a completely different group of foods that upset you. Rather than avoid lots of different items, remove only one food at a time and note any improvements. If you're sure that you really are sensitive to a particular food, try eating smaller amounts of it less often rather than eliminating it altogether. Only remove the food completely from your diet if you're absolutely certain it's the only option.

Before you consider food exclusion, introduce as much of the information provided in this chapter as you can and also check out the section If You Do Nothing Else . . . (see page 250).

Try some rescue remedies

- Onions may be a major cause of gas for some people but onion water can be a very effective remedy. Cut a thin slice of onion, and dip it into a glass of warm water for about ten to fifteen seconds (use water that has been allowed to boil and cool). Remove the onion and then take a sip of the water every hour. This remedy was first given to me at a lecture on herbal medicine in Switzerland and also appears in a brilliant book called *The Nature Doctor* by Dr H.C.A. Vogel.

- The herb savory makes a delicious flavouring added to recipes that contain vegetables, onions or beans, and helps in a major way to reduce wind.

- Diluted peppermint water is another age-old but efficient remedy for ghastly gas.

- Herbal supplements that contain meadowsweet can be very effective non-drug remedies for reducing gas and easing digestive discomfort. Try Potters Acidosis tablets or Meadowsweet & Aniseed from Kiwiherb.

- Charcoal tablets (from a chemist, or try Arkocaps Vegetable Charcoal capsules) are an old-fashioned but effective gas reliever.

- Blackmores Celloid Mineral Sodiphos Compound can reduce bloating by regulating the production of stomach juices, and helping liver function by aiding the digestion of fatty foods and alcohols.

- A quiet spell of relaxation, some deep breathing and abdominal massage (get your partner to rub your tum or do it for yourself) can help to speed relief. And massaging the feet, especially the ball and arch of each foot, or the palms of the hands, can be an effective remedy for some people.

Take a course of digestive enzymes

This is another way to help improve the way your body assimilates its food supply. Take one enzyme with lunch and one with your evening meal. Try Biocare Digestaid, Digestive Enzyme Tablets from Solgar, G&G Digestive Complex, Udo's Choice Digestive Enzyme Blend (Savant) or Viridian Digestive Aid. **Caution: note that digestive enzymes are not suitable if you have gastritis, reflux or ulcers**.

Invest in a course of probiotics

Bloating and gas can be due to a deficiency of good bugs in the bowel. It's also known that the friendly *Lactobacillus acidophilus* helps to alleviate the bloating caused by lactose malabsorption. See page 294 for important probiotic information.

Introduce food combining into your eating plan

When you stop mixing starches with proteins, the improvements in digestion and reduction in bloating can be quite astonishing. Page 283 is the place to find out more.

Bloating can be a problem symbol in a number of other conditions. For more information see candida page 65; diverticular disease page 105; irritable bowel syndrome page 195.

Reducing the risk of bloating

KATHRYN'S TOP TEN TIPS

1. Avoid cow's milk.

2. Avoid sugar.

3. Don't talk while eating.

4. Chew every mouthful really thoroughly.

5. Take more time over meals.

6. Avoid fizzy drinks.

7. Give up the gum.

8. Drink plenty of still (uncarbonated) water between meals.

9. Take a course of probiotics.

10. Practise food combining.

8.

What's Up?
Candida/Thrush

❝ Taking anti-fungal medicine for candida overgrowth without addressing
the underlying reasons for the condition itself "is like trying to weed
your garden by simply cutting the weeds instead of pulling them out by
the roots." ❞

Encyclopaedia of Natural Medicine, Michael T. Murray N.D.
and Joseph E. Pizzorno N.D., 2002

**Read this chapter if you think you have candidiasis or thrush,
or any of the following:**

- Leaky gut syndrome (LGS)
- Food allergies/sensitivities
- Intestinal parasites

You've seen what yeast does to beer or bread. Well, it can do the same
to your digestive system. A major perpetrator of the gas-distended
abdomen is overgrowth of a yeast organism called *Candida albicans*. Every-
body 'has candida'; it's a harmless inhabitant of the intestines. In a healthy
gut, the fungus is kept in check by friendly intestinal flora. But if certain
conditions allow this normally benign yeast to change its form, it runs riot
and creates a very long list of extremely unpleasant symptoms. Damage
occurs only when the normal ecology (symbiosis) of the bowel is disturbed, allowing the yeast to proliferate. At its most troublesome, candida
competes with the bowel's microflora, placing huge strain on the body's

defences. Once changed from Dr Jekyll into Mr Hyde, the yeasty beastie can then 'attack' the healthy membrane between the digestive tract and the bloodstream (or cause further breaches in an already damaged gut wall). Toxic waste products seep into the general circulation, in their turn disrupting the healthy functioning of almost any part of the body.

Don't despair if you're a sufferer. Even if you haven't found help so far, there's plenty of qualified, practical advice available.

What does it all mean?

- *Candida albicans* is the name of the yeast fungus itself. If you see the term *Monilia albicans* anywhere, that's just another label for the same fungus that inhabits the comfy creases and crevices of the gastro-intestinal tract and vaginal tract.

- Thrush (sometimes also referred to by doctors as candidosis), is the common name for the same yeast – but in this case it usually thrives in more visible areas such as the mouth, throat, groin or genitalia. Thrush is usually most people's first clash with *Candida albicans* and is often a result of taking antibiotics that may have been prescribed for acne or an infection following a cold – and very often for cystitis. Although unpleasant and uncomfortable, at this 'surface' level both the cystitis and the thrush should be relatively easy to treat naturally – with diet and immune-boosting nutrients – without resorting to repeat prescriptions of antibiotics. However, the common and constantly repeating cycle of cystitis >> antibiotics >> thrush >> cystitis >> antibiotics is likely to weaken the immune system and drive the yeast 'underground', especially if there are other underlying health problems. Paradoxically, when *Candida albicans* has taken a firm grip on the gut, it may be the case for some people that thrush appears to clear up, only to return to the surface as the system is cleansed and healing begins to take place.

- Candidiasis is a term used by candida specialists to describe the yeast overgrowth that invades and affects the whole body. It's this condition I'll be looking at in more detail in this chapter.

- The word 'candida' is often used as an abbreviation for both the yeast and the condition it causes – probably because it's easier to say than 'candidiasis'.

Medical scepticism

Despite considerable and growing evidence, most allopathic doctors still don't accept the existence of the condition. While they agree upon the existence of vaginal and oral thrush (and on chronic systemic candidiasis in patients suffering terminal illness), many remain resistant to the idea that this 'harmless' yeast could otherwise create such internal havoc. As a result, most medical dictionaries and the majority of doctors still use the terms candidosis, candidiasis and thrush to mean the same thing – fungal infection at a superficial or surface level.

Candidiasis may appear to be a relatively new condition but actually it isn't. As long ago as 1931, doctors researching an illness with almost identical problems coined the phrase 'carbohydrate dyspepsia' to describe collective symptoms such as gas, bowel discomfort, irritable bladder, bloating, muscle pain and unexplained fatigue. Treatment involved the restriction of sweet and starchy foods, and supplementation of pancreatic enzymes, probiotics and vitamins – not dissimilar to today's recommendations.

In the late 1970s, Dr C. Orian Truss presented research suggesting that a common mould, *Candida albicans*, could be the trigger for an almost identical set of symptoms which he classified under the general heading of 'dysfunctional gut syndrome'. However, as far as orthodox science was concerned, the concept of a 'physical' cause remained 'unproven'. Conventional medicine took the view that most symptoms were 'probably psychiatric in origin'. But listening to sufferers as well as to the practitioners who specialise in treating their condition, it seems unlikely in the extreme that candidiasis is 'all in the mind'.

The symptoms

Symptoms associated with candidiasis include:

Aching	Cramp
Allergies	Cravings
Anxiety	Cystitis
Bloating	Depression
Bowel problems	Digestive discomfort
Chronic fatigue	Dizziness

Dry cough	Nausea
Flatulence	Palpitations
Food sensitivities	Persistent infections
Gas	Poor concentration
Headaches or migraine	Poor coordination
Hypoglycaemia	Poor immunity to infections
Impaired recall	Premenstrual syndrome
Irritability	Rectal itching
Irritable bowel	Skin eruptions
Lack of energy	'Spaced out' feelings
Lethargy	Stiff joints
Loss of – or low – libido	Thrush
Menstrual problems	Vaginal dryness
Mood swings	Vaginal irritation
Muscle pain	Weight gain

As you can see, the list of symptoms is long – and this isn't all of them! The presence of *Candida albicans* can itself aggravate and perpetrate a number of other conditions. including migraine, hypoglycaemia, acne, eczema, psoriasis, urticaria, hyperactivity, premenstrual syndrome, asthma, food allergies, ear infections, hypothyroidism, irritable bowel syndrome and chronic fatigue syndrome (ME). Moreover, many of the symptoms are similar to a number of other digestive dysfunctions, including food sensitivity and leaky gut syndrome, making it impossible to work out which came first. No wonder it's so easy to miss – or to misdiagnose. It's for this reason that I always recommend anyone who suspects they might be suffering from candidiasis to see a specialist who is familiar with the nutritional treatment of this complex condition. Page 222 has more on leaky gut syndrome and page 115 more on allergies.

Who can get candidiasis?

Candidiasis can affect anyone at any age but is believed to be around eight times more likely to occur in women than in men, because it's aggravated by the birth control pill, hormone replacement therapy (HRT) and increased numbers of antibiotic prescriptions for cystitis.

The likely triggers can include:

Adrenal exhaustion
Antibiotics
Contraceptive pill
Corticosteroid drugs
Depressed immunity
Diets high in sugar
Environmental and chemical overload
Excess alcohol
Hormone replacement therapy
Imbalance of friendly gut flora
Immune suppressing drugs
Inadequate levels of digestive enzymes
Low thyroid function
Non-steroidal anti-inflammatory drugs (NSAIDs)
Poor liver function
Poor-quality diet/inadequate nutrients
Protracted negative stress

Of all the things on this list, certainly from my own practice experience, depressed immunity has to be the major factor in the explosion of candidiasis. According to leading candida specialist Sherridan Stock: 'a weak immune system appears to be the norm these days, the main reason for which, in our opinion, is nutrient deficiency. Almost every nutrient known has a role to play in creating immunity, and since most individuals exhibit multiple nutrient deficiencies, they inevitably have chronically impaired immune systems.'

The body can't cope

I see the rise of candidiasis also depending very much on 'overload'. In other words, a properly nourished body may be well equipped to manage short periods of stress, exhaustion, illness, chemical exposure, and so on. Add frequent courses of antibiotics to, say, a diet high in sugar and lacking in dietary fibre, drop in a few viruses or heavy doses of petrochemical fumes for good measure, pile on the stress and ignore the need for rest, sleep and nourishing food, and you are well on the way to breaking point. Every detrimental move makes it easier for *Candida albicans* to escalate and intensify.

Action plan for candidiasis/thrush

Encouragingly, an increasing number of nutritionally aware doctors are accepting the presence of candidiasis and are willing to treat it. To be successful, treatment requires a several-pronged 'annihilate and nurture' programme. In other words, kill off the invasive yeast with anti-fungal supplements, heal the gut and boost the immune system to protect against further attack. Isolated use of anti-fungal drugs without addressing the underlying factors may result only in short-term improvements. In any event, candidiasis is not a condition that you should attempt to cope with alone, without experience and knowledge. It's a complex problem, necessitating a full clinical evaluation by an experienced and qualified practitioner who is familiar with the nutritional treatment of candidiasis. Ask about the tests that are available to check for candida and parasites. If your practitioner is not aware of them or cannot offer this service, I would seriously consider finding another practitioner.

Please don't launch into a restricted dietary regime because you think that, by avoiding long lists of different foods, your candidiasis will give up the ghost. It's unlikely this approach will work. There may be short-term relief, but drastic dietary measures are far more likely to lead to worsening deficiencies and consequent malnourishment. Poor immunity and lack of nutrients are two of the most likely reasons why *Candida albicans* picked on you in the first place. So don't cut calories. Eating healthily and well is essential to full recovery. Apart from the suggestions that follow, leave the initial guidance on foods to a nutritionist.

Some self-help

Here are some important steps that you can take while you are waiting to see a practitioner.

Your diet

Avoid all sugar and sugary foods

Because *Candida albicans* absolutely adores sugar, it's well accepted that strict sugar avoidance is an absolute priority for anyone who is serious about treating the condition. Feedback suggests that the majority of people experience significant improvements simply by avoiding added and hidden sugar (and, at least during treatment, that includes syrups, honey and fruit juices).

Don't use artificial sweeteners

They are not an acceptable sugar substitute. In the case of chronic candidiasis, these chemicals are merely another straw to the overloaded liver and underfunctioning digestive system.

Get into the food combining habit

It really does seem to help reduce candida symptoms, not for everyone but certainly for the vast majority of sufferers. Forget my views – they're bound to be biased. But I can tell you that feedback from other practitioners and from former patients is very positive. A good place to start finding out about this would be my book *The Complete Book of Food Combining* or *Food Combining In 30 Days*. (Try your local bookshop, library or ordering online.)

Drink more water

Drink more – preferably filtered water (see Chapter 24).

Take cold-pressed aloe vera juice

Do this every day. Add half a cup (approximately 60 millilitres) to a glass of organic cranberry juice. Try Xynergy Health or Higher Nature for really good-quality aloe vera products.

Cut out cow's milk

Make sure you avoid ordinary cow's milk completely and absolutely. The high lactose content of cow's milk promotes the growth of *Candida albicans*. And, unless it's organic, it may contain traces of antibiotics that can further disrupt the levels of friendly flora and promote more yeast. Sheep's or goat's milk yoghurt can be a valuable substitute unless you are intolerant of all dairy products. Organic soya milk, oat milk and Rice Dream are useful non-dairy alternatives. My 'swap box' starting on page 251 has more ideas.

Avoid yeast drinks and foods

Cut out alcoholic beverages, breads and other baked goods and anything containing yeast. Adding dietary yeast to the body simply encourages your candida.

Eat the freshest possible foods

Always check the 'use-by' date on everything you buy and make sure it's consumed well within that date. Foods that readily attract mould can be a particular hazard for candida sufferers since moulds are well-known allergy triggers and can put further pressure on an already leaky or inflamed gut.

Steer clear of suspect foods

All the items in the following list are frequently claimed by candida sufferers to aggravate their symptoms. While you're waiting to see a practitioner, I'd strongly suggest that if you do eat anything from this list it's absolutely fresh, and that you only eat it in minimum quantities.

Canned and cartoned juices
Canned foods, especially tomato products (check labels – most have
    added sugar)
Cheeses
Cold cuts of meat
Dried fruits
Foods containing citric acid (especially oranges, grapefruits and lemons)
Herbs, chilli and curry
Mayonnaise, salad cream, foods containing vinegar
Mushrooms
Nuts
Peanuts
Pickles and relishes
Sauerkraut
Smoked fish
Smoked, preserved meats
Soy sauce
Stock cubes and yeast extracts such as Marmite
Syrups and honey
White rice (brown is usually fine but must be freshly cooked)

Watch the fresh fruit

Fruit can aggravate symptoms in some sufferers simply because of its natural sugar content. However, fruit is also a nutritious food and if you gave it up altogether you'd be losing out on a lot of valuable nourishment. So the following tips may be helpful. During the early stages of treatment I'd suggest that if you include fresh fruit:

- Make sure it is really very fresh.

- Limit yourself to one piece per day.

- Bypass any fruit that is very ripe or over-ripe.

- Eat fruit on an empty stomach; it can be easier to digest if eaten this way.

Avoid fruit completely if you find that it causes symptoms to flare.

Check labels for the 'H' word

Swap all *hydrogenated* margarines for non-hydrogenated alternatives (from health food stores). And change polyunsaturated cooking oils for extra-virgin olive oil. Don't be conned into thinking that 'margarine-type' spreads made with olive oil are going to be as healthy as the oil itself. It's unlikely to be true.

Use cold-pressed nut and seed oils

These can include flax, pumpkin seed, hemp, extra-virgin and safflower oils. This is a useful way of taking in nutritious omega 3 and 6 essential fatty acids, which are lacking in the majority of diets. An excellent choice for candida sufferers is Udo's Choice Ultimate Oil Blend (from Savant) which, in addition to flax, sunflower, sesame and evening primrose oils, contains coconut oil, a source of anti-fungal caprylic acid. Other high-quality oil options include those from Green People, Arkopharma, Viridian and Higher Nature. Use these special oils for drizzling onto vegetables and salads, and add them to soups and juices. Never heat them. For use as spreads, nut or seed butters such as almond, cashew, hazelnut or pumpkin butter are nourishing alternatives to dairy butter.

Eat plain bio-yoghurt daily

If possible, choose yoghurt made from sheep's or goat's milk or soya. Health food stores are probably your most likely source of supply. Some supermarkets are willing to put in a special order if you buy from them regularly. Don't be put off if you don't like the first brand you try. Some sheep's and goat's milk yoghurts can seem sharp compared to creamy cow's milk varieties, but other labels (St Helen's Dairy & Woodlands Park Dairy for example) are smooth and delicious. There is also a sheep's milk version of the Total Greek Yoghurt available in most major supermarkets. Check the label carefully.

Take certain supplements

The following might be helpful:

- Digestive enzymes taken with your lunch and evening meal. See page 267 for more information.

- Natural anti-fungal supplements. Oregano oil is a particularly effective anti-fungal agent. Other plant extracts, such as peppermint, rosemary, goldenseal, thyme, clove, wormwood, barberry and black walnut, are all used in various combinations to help reduce yeasts, toxins, parasites and bacteria. Always choose top-quality products from recognised suppliers. See Resource Directory (page 323) for details.

- Always including echinacea. Although, on its own, this herb does not have a great deal of anti-fungal activity, echinacea's major benefit seems to be that it works on candidiasis by helping to boost the immune system. Several different brands are available, as tablets, capsules or tinctures, from health food stores, some chemists and larger supermarkets. Top of my list are Bioforce Echinaforce Drops, Biocare Echinacea Capsules, Blackmores Echinacea, Viridian Organic Echinacea Tincture and Echinacea Root Extract from Kiwi Herb.

- Going for garlic. As long as you are not allergic to garlic, add it to your cooking, grate it raw into salads and over vegetables or, if you don't like the taste of it in your food, try it as a supplement. It's a fabulous anti-fungal so, even if you're not keen on garlic, be comforted by the fact that candida really loathes it. I would suggest using Garlic Plus from Biocare or Blackmores Garlix Tablets. They're definitely not odourless but, I believe, are more effective than the deodorised brands. Take your daily garlic supplement in the middle of a meal to lessen the risk of it 'repeating'.

- Including a detoxifying fibre supplement such as psyllium husk or linseeds in your daily diet. Page 27 has the low-down on high fibre and product recommendations.

VERY IMPORTANT POINT

Supplements should never be considered a substitute for healthy foods. However, if you live in an area of the world where it's difficult to obtain organic foods or where fresh foods are in short supply, it's all the more important to source top-quality supplements, especially probiotics, which are always available by mail order. The Resource Directory (see page 323) has contact details.

What else can you do?

Cut your exposure to chemicals

These include artificial food additives and pesticides. Buy natural cosmetics, household cleaning materials and bath products. Choose bleach-free panti-pads. Avoid processed, packaged foods as much as possible – they're usually heavily laced with artificial additives. Don't use artificial sweeteners. Make every effort to steer clear of cigarette smoke – yours and other people's. Don't exercise near a busy road. And fit an air purifier to your car (see Resource Directory, page 323).

Take care with moulds

If household mould appears on any surface, never 'dry wipe' it as this can scatter the spores. Wipe it away with an anti-fungal solution and remove the clean moisture with a dry cloth afterwards. Diluted bleach or household disinfectant works well but may be an additional source of chemical allergy. Diluted bicarbonate of soda can be an effective mould killer, as is Borax. I usually use a few drops of tea tree oil or Manuka oil (New

Zealand tea tree oil) sloshed around in a bowl of water if I want to clean and disinfect any non-polished surfaces.

Treat for Giardia lamblia

Symptoms of this prolific parasite, which is transmitted through contaminated water and by sexual contact, cleverly mimic many of the symptoms of candidiasis – and those of chronic fatigue syndrome. Page 177 contains more information about intestinal parasites. Please read it even if you don't think you're affected.

Consider the probability of other conditions

There are various other health problems that have symptoms very similar to those of candidiasis; for example, leaky gut syndrome and food allergy (as well as *Giardia lamblia* mentioned above). If the symptoms I've described in this chapter seem to describe just what you are going through, then in addition to seeking professional practitioner support I would also suggest that you check out the chapters on food allergy (see page 115) and leaky gut syndrome (see page 222), which may also be relevant.

Take the load off your liver

A simple detox can be a real holiday for this hard-working organ. I don't have the space here to describe detoxification in detail so can I suggest that you obtain a copy of my book, *The Complete Book of Food Combining*, and read pages 202–249. Good supplements to assist detox include Milk Thistle tablets (Solgar, Viridian, Bio-Health, Blackmores), Sodium Sulphate (Blackmores) and Bioforce Detox Box.

Think positively, deal with stress and get plenty of rest

Negative thinking, stress and lack of sleep put further pressure on the immune system.

Talk to your doctor

Discuss any medication you are taking with your doctor and check to see if it is really essential. Antibiotics are an obvious problem, but did you know that some anti-ulcer drugs can encourage the growth of *Candida albicans* in the stomach?

Massage your abdomen

Do this with a little olive oil or olive oil cream every day. First thing in the morning or last thing at night are the best times. Pay particular attention to your ileo-caecal valve (see below).

Helpful hint

Locate your ileo-caecal valve (ICV)
It's just inside the right hip bone, near to the appendix. This junction between the small and large intestines tends to suffer from poor muscle tone, allowing back-flow of bacteria and poisonous wastes and a build-up of toxicity. Not only do the symptoms of autointoxication, which result from a faulty ICV (headaches, lethargy, aching, dizziness, bloating, nausea and other digestive disturbance), bear a close resemblance to those of chronic candidiasis, but it's also likely that a defective ICV could exacerbate a candida condition and vice versa. Indeed, leading practitioners in the treatment of candidiasis believe that the two conditions of small bowel toxicity and overgrowth of *Candida albicans* often coexist. Practised regularly, abdominal massage (see box, page 78) helps to tone the muscles and strengthen the IC valve.

Snippets
By the way, the term 'autointoxication' was first coined by Dr Eli Metchnikoff in his book *The Prolongation of Life* (G.P. Putnam 1908) to describe what happens when harmful toxins, produced by disease-promoting bacteria, are absorbed into the bloodstream. Although the word has nothing to do with being three sheets to the wind or in any way the worse for drink, I think it describes well a digestive system that is very definitely 'under the weather'.

A Simple Massage

Help to reduce candida symptoms by doing this simple massage every day:

Lie on a bed or long sofa (you need to be lying flat and stretched out). Make sure that you're comfortable. Remove sufficient clothing so that your abdomen is exposed. Cover your legs and torso with blankets or towels to make sure that you stay as warm as possible. To massage, use one teaspoon of either extra-virgin olive oil or pumpkin seed oil. If you have them available, mix one drop of essential oil of rosemary and one drop of fennel with the base oil before use. These oils are soothing if you have digestive discomfort or bloating.

Beginning just inside the right hip bone, at the IC valve, near to where the top of the leg meets the groin, use the pads of your fingers to massage your abdomen. Work your way up the right-hand side towards the waist, across the belly, over to the left-hand side and down again until you are level with the left hip bone. Then massage, left to right, across the middle of the abdomen, and back again so that the whole of the area is covered.

Tip: If you don't have strong fingers or have arthritis in your finger joints, it may be more comfortable to use the flat of your hand to massage.

Recommended reading

Read Jane McWhirter's excellent book, *The Practical Guide To Candida*. It costs £11, including postage, and is available direct from 01621 810323, or send cheque with order to 93 Ram Gorse, Harlow, Essex CM20 1PZ. All proceeds from the book go to the health charity, The All Hallows Foundation for Education and Research. You also might be interested in the video *Clear From Candida*. It is comprehensive and detailed, with a three-hour running time. The cost is £21, including postage. Make your cheque payable to Candida Workshops and send your order to Gibliston Mill, Colinsburgh, Leven, Fife KY9 1JS. Also worthwhile and available from booksellers is *Beat Candida Through Diet* by Gill Jacobs.

Reducing the risk of candidiasis

KATHRYN'S TOP TEN TIPS

1. Follow a diet rich in fresh vegetables and salads.

2. Use as much organic produce as you can.

3. Get into the food-combining habit.

4. Keep sugar, yeast and alcohol intake to a minimum.

5. Avoid cow's milk.

6. Reduce chemical exposure.

7. Follow a regular two-day detox.

8. Use garlic in your cooking and take garlic supplements.

9. Follow a three-month course of probiotics every twelve months and always take probiotics after completing a course of antibiotics.

10. Check out the book and website details that follow.

WWW

www.candida-society.org.uk is the site for the National Candida Society, Box 151, Orpington, Kent BR5 1UJ. Inexpensive annual membership gives you regular newsletters, a helpline and local support. Send a stamped addressed envelope to P.O. Box 151, Orpington, Kent BR5 1UJ.
www.chemicalbodyburden.org is a useful reference if you're concerned, as we all should be, about the overload of chemicals in our diet and environment.

9.

What's Up?
Constipation

> **Read this chapter if you are suffering from constipation, or think you may be suffering from:**
>
> - Irritable bowel syndrome (IBS)
> - Diverticulitis
> - Haemorrhoids (piles)

Perhaps it would help if governments took a more open and relaxed view of bowel disease. Twenty thousand people are lost each year through bowel cancer and yet, in the UK Government's own strategy document *The Health of the Nation*, which was supposedly planned to help us all towards better health, there is – at the time of writing this book – not one word of advice on the subject.

I would say that this is possibly one of the most important sections in the whole book. It has vital links to conditions discussed in other sections, and I do hope you'll read it.

What exactly is constipation?

Constipation is your body's way of letting you know that something isn't right. It's defined in medical terminology as 'unduly infrequent and difficult evacuation, usually of hard, dry faeces'. The most likely causes include a diet lacking in sufficient fibre or fluid, lack of exercise or the deliberate suppression of the urge to 'go'. Simple constipation is an incredibly common condition and almost always easy to treat. But it can be the cause of many other ailments, some of them potentially very serious.

The constipated personality

Attitude to life can be a causative factor in constipation. If we're always rushing and never have time to do things for ourselves, we are also likely to say we're too busy for bodily functions. If we postpone bathroom stops because we think it will help us to make up lost time, the chances are that our intestines will be as clogged as the journey home through rush-hour traffic on a Friday afternoon.

If we accumulate emotional baggage, we may also be holding on to physical baggage. Unwillingness to discuss or display our *e-motions* may connect with a similar reluctance to let go of our *motions*. This won't apply to everyone who has constipation but, in my experience with patients, it has been a frequent finding. Colleagues are aware of similar case histories. Fear of letting go of faeces can mean we hold on to hurt and don't want to face the consequences of past unhappiness or resentment. In the same way that poisons from a compacted colon are reabsorbed into the bloodstream, stored sadness or mean memories can recirculate too, poisoning our minds. Sometimes, it's almost as if the ability never to forget some unpleasant event long past is the sufferer's security – a way of keeping information that could be held against the original perpetrator.

The real sadness of this is that, in most cases, the event was trivial and probably long forgotten by everyone else. One of the keys to overcoming constipation could be to let go of the past and to forgive the person who caused you the pain. This doesn't mean that you have to condone their behaviour, but you can simply eliminate the sorrow and accept that:

a) whatever it was that happened, happened,

b) it isn't healthy to hold on to it and

c) you don't need it anymore.

Don't ignore it

Constipation left untreated may – literally – have grave consequences. Research confirms that those who suffer persistent constipation have a greater risk of contracting bowel cancer in later life than those who don't. There are also several other serious diseases that can have chronic constipation as a major symptom. These include neurological disorders and anything that affects the nervous system, such as Parkinson's disease, spinal cord injuries, diabetes or stroke, muscular disorders, chronic intestinal obstructions, problems with liver function, the kidneys, pancreas or thyroid, structural changes (surgery) and hormonal disorders.

Conditions such as bloating, digestive discomfort, hiatus hernia and headaches can have a variety of likely causes. One of them could be – you guessed it – constipation. People who have suffered from constipation for years may never consider that their permanent state of general unwellness could be due entirely to their compacted colon. Constipation is a major factor in haemorrhoids and in diverticular disease, and can aggravate a hiatus hernia. Acne and eczema-like skin eruptions can be a sign that toxins from a silted colon have been reabsorbed into the bloodstream.

Occasionally, some people with constipation don't respond to standard treatment. When doctors can't find a reason for constipation, they call it chronic idiopathic constipation (which means it's of unknown origin).

Likely causes or triggers

These include:

Ageing
Digestive enzyme deficiency
Diverticular disease
Hiatus hernia
Irritable bowel syndrome
Laxatives – especially if they are used too frequently
Lack of dietary fibre
Lack of exercise
Nervous tension

Not drinking enough water
Piles (haemorrhoids)
Poor muscle tone
Poor liver or gall-bladder function
Pregnancy
Prostate problems
Some drug medications, including codeine, antidepressants, diuretics,
    antihypertensives, muscle relaxants, iron supplements, steroids, antibiotics
    and non-steroidal anti-inflammatory drugs (NSAIDs).

Likely symptoms

The likely symptoms include the following:

Acid reflux	Haemorrhoids
Anal fissures	Irritable bowel
Bad breath	Reduced appetite
Bloated abdomen	Nausea
Body odour	Smelly feet
Cramp	Skin problems
Coated tongue	Sluggishness
Fatigue	Wind pain
Headaches	

Other problems?

- Constipation may cause the sufferer to urinate more frequently because of pressure against the bladder.

- Bowel movements may occur in response to the release of bile from the gall bladder. If the liver and gall bladder are sluggish, the bowel may not receive the right messages and wastes will, literally, back up.

- Intermittent patches of diarrhoea can be a symptom of constipation. If old faeces harden against the colon wall, new wastes can't make contact. Water doesn't get reabsorbed and the faeces remain semi-liquid. Result? Diarrhoea. Similarly, if a solidified stool has lodged in the rectum or further up in the sigmoid colon, liquid wastes that haven't had a chance to form properly into the usual shaped blobs will have no other option but to 'leak' their way past the blockage. Called faecal impaction, this is most common in children and in the elderly and is usually treated with a laxative that lubricates or softens the stool, helping it to break up and be passed more easily.

- Bright red blood in the stools can indicate the presence of piles but may also be a sign of an anal fissure, a small tear in the anal membrane caused by straining when stools are hard to pass.

Straining can sometimes cause a small amount of the intestine's lining to push out into the anal opening. Known as rectal prolapse, the first sign may be a leakage of mucus from the anus. Severe prolapse requires surgery.

Have you opened your bowels today?

For most people, 'once a day' seems quite normal. For others, every few days might be their 'regular' pattern. Even doctors can't agree on an ideal frequency. Some say that there is no right or wrong number of daily bowel movements, and that 'normal' can be three times a day or three times a week. Others experts, including naturopathic and nutrition specialists, believe that twelve hours is a healthier transit time of food from entrance to exit – in other words, twice daily. It's generally agreed that if your stools are soft and easy to pass then you are unlikely to be constipated. If they're hard and difficult to get rid of – and you're going fewer than three times a week – then that constitutes constipation.

Did you know?
Despite high levels of national constipation, it's estimated that the United Kingdom uses some 1,500,000,000 toilet rolls every year.

Unfortunately, our not-so-great eating habits and lifestyle stresses can very easily reduce our regular bathroom visits to intervals of seventy-two or more hours. It's not unusual to see patients who admit to 'going' only once a fortnight! And if you think that's bad, consider the world constipation record, which was once claimed to be 102 days!

Every now and then, we all suffer from backed-up solids. A change of diet or a change of scene, such as being away from home, are the most likely causes. Getting back into a normal routine, and making sure we drink enough fluid, eat a fresh, wholefood diet, and take regular exercise, are nearly always effective remedies for a temporarily sluggish bowel. But what do we do if our constipation is deep rooted and long established?

Did you know?

... why your wastes are brown? The colour of crap is determined mostly by discarded red blood cells and a substance called bilirubin, a constituent of bile. Remember that bile is produced by the liver and stored in the gall bladder, and is used to help the digestion of fats in the diet. But the body also uses bile to help get rid of wastes. So redundant bile gets mixed with other garbage – such as the bilirubin – which eventually finds its way to the large intestine.

See your doctor

- If your constipation is worsening despite all your best efforts.

- If you're unable to have bowel movements without using laxatives.

- If your constipation is accompanied by any kind of severe pain or nausea.

- If you have any uncontrolled leakage of stools.

- If you see blood mixed with your stools. If the blood is dark red or your faeces seem to be streaked with black, see you doctor without delay. Bright red blood is usually a sign of a haemorrhoid or an anal fissure. Dark blood in the stools can indicate bleeding further up the digestive tract, possibly in the stomach. Whatever the cause, continued bleeding can lead to anaemia and could indicate an illness that requires immediate attention.

- You should also tell your doctor:
  - How long constipation has been a problem.
  - What remedies you have tried.

- Whether your faeces are hard, soft or mucusy.
- How often you go to the toilet.
- If there is a history of constipation in the family.
- If there is a history of bowel cancer.

Action plan for constipation

Your diet

Drink more fluid

Increasing the amount that you drink helps make faeces softer and easier to eliminate. This is certainly just as important as increasing your intake of dietary fibre. Unfortunately, alcohol doesn't count in the quota because it doesn't hydrate. Coffee, soda pop and other sweet fizzy drinks tend to be dehydrating, too. Tea, which contains less caffeine, is a better option than coffee. Better still are fresh juices, especially vegetable juices, herbal and fruit teas, soups and, of course, water.

There's no need to feel as if you are drowning in glasses of H_2O. If you drink a glass of water when you first get up in the morning, have juice or tea with breakfast, and take another glass of water before lunch and again before your evening meal, that's already four glasses gone. Add your other usual beverages and count the fluid that comes from the fruits and vegetables you eat each day (see page 289 for information on quantities), and you are well on your way to taking in the right amount of daily fluid.

Increase your intake of fibre

If you've increased your fibre intake already and had no results, consider changing the type of fibre you are using. They're not all the same. I've written up a whole separate section on this subject which you'll find under fibre tips (see page 271) so I'll say no more about it just here.

Eat foods rich in calcium and magnesium

A regular selection from the following list should provide a good balance of these minerals, which are often found lacking in people with constipation.

Magnesium-rich foods include:

Almonds	Garlic
Apples	Ginger root
Bananas	Grapefruit
Brazil nuts	Lamb
Brown rice	Lemons
Cashews	Pasta
Dried fruits, especially figs	Pulses
Fish	Seafood
Fresh fruits	Wholegrains

Calcium-rich foods include:

Almonds	Goat's milk yoghurt and cheese
Blackstrap molasses	Sea vegetables
Brazil nuts	Sesame seeds
Brown rice	Sheep's milk yoghurt and cheese
Buttermilk	Sunflower seeds
Canned sardines, pilchards and salmon	Tofu
Carob flour	The majority of vegetables and herbs contain some calcium.
Dried fruits	A list of some of the best sources
Fortified soya milk	is on page 217.

Avoid potato starch or white flour

Both potato starch and refined wheat starch may cause or aggravate constipation in some sufferers, so try to avoid foods containing them. It may be that the pancreas isn't able to produce enough starch-splitting enzymes to break down these two foods but, in any event, it seems that the starch can have a binding effect in some people. Cold cooked potatoes and jacket potatoes are, on the other hand, good gut foods.

Practise food combining

You may be surprised that something as simple as changing the order or the combination of the foods on your plate could affect how often you go to the lavatory. Nevertheless, food combining does seem to have an extremely beneficial and yet gentle effect on a reluctant colon. See page 283 for more information.

What else can you do?

Get moving

A common cause of constipation is lack of exercise. If you don't do any, your circulation slows down and muscle tone slackens. Not only does this affect the peristaltic contractions of the large intestine, but weak muscles also make defaecation more difficult. There's no need to work out until you drop or spend boring or excessive hours at the gym. Thirty minutes a day is the amount recommended to help maintain a healthy heart. Taking a brisk fifteen-minute walk after lunch and another one later in the day sometimes seems easier and less time consuming.

Housebound or not so mobile? If your constipation is worse as a result of immobility, ask your doctor or practice nurse about the possibility of a consultation with the local physiotherapist who can give you exercises to do at home. Bowels usually become more slothful with age. As activity levels and metabolism slow down, muscle tone is reduced and intestinal movements become sluggish, making constipation a common affliction of the elderly. Even light exercise can make a big difference.

Watch your medication

Some types of medication can cause constipation. If you're already drinking plenty of liquid, you're sure that your dietary fibre intake is good and you're taking plenty of exercise, but constipation is still a problem, talk to your doctor or a pharmacist about the likely side-effects of any medicines you're taking.

Don't rely on laxatives

If you find you are constipated after a change of routine, don't reach automatically for the laxatives. Not only can they be habit forming, but they also make the bowel lazy. They work by irritating the lining of the bowel and, in the long term, can damage nerves and interfere with the natural ability of muscles to contract. Herbal laxatives may be a useful occasional alternative but, like any laxative, they are not designed for long-term use. Always read the label and do not exceed the stated dose. Unless advised specifically not to do so by your medical practitioner, always make sure that you drink plenty of water. Never give laxatives of any kind to children or to the elderly unless under medical prescription and supervision.

Most people who are only mildly constipated are unlikely to need laxatives. If you're unsure, talk to a pharmacist or your doctor. If lifestyle changes and a different diet have made no difference, you may be recommended a laxative preparation. A short course of laxatives can help bring bowel behaviour back to normal. There are several kinds available:

- Fibre supplements, also known as bulking agents, are taken with water and are designed to bulk the stools, making them easier to pass. They are usually made with plant fibre such as bran, sterculia, isphagula (or its close relative psyllium) or with synthetic cellulose.

- Faecal softeners such as liquid paraffin and the drug docusate sodium do just what the name suggests. They soften the stools, easing straining. They are often prescribed where there are painful rectal conditions such as piles or fissures.

- Stimulant laxatives like senna or bisacodyl trigger the muscular contractions needed to move wastes along.

- Osmotic laxatives draw water into the colon, again softening the stools. One of the best-known laxatives in this category is lactulose. Polyethylene glycol is usually used to clean the colon before colonoscopy. Glycerol suppositories are a gentle treatment, especially useful where fibrous or other supplements may not be suitable, for example for the elderly.

Get to the root of the problem

Make every effort to suss out the cause of your constipation and then resolve to make the necessary changes. There is absolutely no point in living or eating just any old way and then trying to overcome the discomforts by half-hearted or occasional improvements to your diet, the odd clean-up or a load of laxatives.

> **Helpful hint**
> If you need a little help, try one of these remedies with a glass of water. They all contain good sources of dietary fibre.
>
> - **Linseeds** (read important information on linseeds, page 278).
> - **Psyllium husks** (powder or tablets) available from health food stores, or check stockist information (see page 323).
> - Three or four **dried figs or soaked prunes**, chewed thoroughly.
>
> **Very important and worth saying again: always accompany any kind of fibre with a glass of water.**

Take vitamin C

I've found that vitamin C taken before meals can help to improve regularity. Ask in your health food store or look out for good brands such as Blackmores, Viridian, Solgar, Biocare and Bioforce. Follow the pack instructions and don't take more than the recommended dose. Avoid those large tablets, usually available from the chemist, that dissolve in water; they can be very acidic and may upset a sensitive digestion.

Improve your digestion

Anything you do to improve the way your body handles its food should be good for your colon too. Check out the chapter If You Do Nothing Else . . . (see page 250).

Deal with anxiety and stress

Are you a tight, taut person who lives on your nerves? Restlessness, anxiety and constant hurrying can have a detrimental effect on the nervous system. Changing pace and bringing some tranquillity and calmness into your life is as important as any diet or exercise.

If you are really struggling against the tide and stress is completely invading your life, talk to your doctor or practice nurse and tell them how you feel. Bowel disorders can often be triggered by emotional rather than physical upset or worry. There may be a problem, either now or in your past, that could be causing you to 'hold on' to baggage or to be afraid of 'letting go' – something that, perhaps, you aren't even aware of. Anxiety, inability to relax and the negative effects of stress can all contribute to constipation. This doesn't mean that your bowel problems aren't real, but simply that there may be causes other than obvious ones that might be aggravating the symptoms.

Try some supplements

The following might help:

- Bowel Essence, one of the Jan de Vries Flower Essences, can be helpful if your gut is gripped by emotional upset or excessive stress. I've also heard really good reports of an Arkopharma product, Californian Poppy, helping to relieve stress-related constipation.

- The herb milk thistle, taken at mealtimes, may be a useful supplement if your constipation is caused by a lethargic liver. Bio-Health, Blackmores, Solgar and Viridian are good brands to look out for. Blackmores Sodiphos Compound is also useful for improving liver function and helping in the detoxification process. If you suffer from long-term constipation that seems resistant to dietary changes, the Bioforce Detox Box is well worth trying.

- Change of routine? If your bowels have seized up as a result of you being away from home or for some reason not getting enough dietary fibre, a good-quality fibre supplement in tablet or capsule form can be a boon. Blackmores and Biocare both make a product called Colon Care. Take with a glass of water two or three times a day, just before meals.

Massage your abdomen

See page 78 for an explanation of this soothing, comforting and often very effective remedy.

Try toilet training

Pay attention to your bowels

Don't get emotional about your motions but do try to understand a little about how your body works and respond to your gut's intelligence. Go when you feel the need. When your bowel wants to empty, it sends you a message to tell you so. So if you receive a sign that you need to visit the lavatory, answer the call. However busy you are, don't let your bowel go back to sleep.

Make time for it

Your health depends upon it. The longer you leave it, the larger and more solid the solids become, as more and more toxins are going to be absorbed. Ignoring the urge to empty your bowels can cause the feedback mechanisms to switch off so that eventually you stop feeling the urge. On the infrequent occasions when you do go, wastes are rough, hard, dry and painful. It's no accident that constipation has been likened to 'passing bricks'. Procrastinating not only increases the risk of constipation, cramping and bloating, but could also lead to even more serious bowel disorders.

Go after meals

Some practitioners recommend visiting the toilet twenty minutes after each meal (whether or not you feel the need to go) as this can help establish a natural reflex to open the bowels. If nothing else, it's one way of escaping for a period of quiet meditation! Just don't take the portable telephone with you! Return any calls when you're free or let the caller ring you again.

Don't strain

Be patient. You may live in a world that demands everything yesterday, but don't push your body into performing instant defecation. Straining only increases the risk of piles and anal fissures, and weakens the muscles in the bowel wall.

Practise the pelvic squeeze

First introduced by Dr Arnold Kegel in 1948 to help patients suffering from stress incontinence, these exercises improve blood flow to the pelvic area and strengthen the muscles that support the bladder, rectum and anal sphincter. Done regularly, they can reduce the tendency to strain and prevent the loss of accidental waste; they are helpful if you're prone to either constipation or urgent diarrhoea. They're also known to enhance vaginal sensitivity and lubrication. Tighten up as if you were trying to stop yourself 'spending a penny'. Hold for two or three seconds and then relax. Squeeze, hold and let go. Repeat ten times at each session.

Correct technique is important so it can help to read an inexpensive booklet (and a world best-seller, so it shows how common this problem is) on 'Kegels' before you begin. *Women's Waterworks* by Dr Pauline Chiarelli is available from www.winhealth.co.uk, telephone 01835 864 866, fax 01835 863 238. There are also pelvic toners/vaginal exercisers available that can improve the results you get from doing Kegel exercises. Pay for a good-quality product. Cheap ones are not usually worth the money. You can obtain information – including a really useful leaflet called *Improve Your Pelvic Health* – from www.natural-woman.com or call 0117 968 7744.

Don't concentrate too hard

Bowels have a funny habit of switching off if you pay them too much attention. Take something to read or let your mind wander. Concentrating on anything but the matter in hand can help to relax you.

Resort to books

Take a couple of large books with you (big reference works such as a dictionary and an encyclopedia are ideal), one to put under each foot. This repositioning of the legs helps to relax the muscles that are used during defaecation and mimics the more natural near-squatting position. If you don't have suitable books, try putting your feet on an upturned washing-up bowl, low footstool or other similarly shaped object, but make sure it's firm and not likely to slip, and that you push any foot supports out of the way and put your feet firmly back down on the floor before standing up.

Lift one foot and then the other

While you're sitting, waiting for things to happen, try 'walking up and down on the spot', so to speak. Just raise one foot from the floor and put it down again. Then do the same with the other foot. This is another action that helps to relax the muscles in the rectum and around the anal sphincter. Try coordinating the movements with your breathing. Breathe in as you lift the foot up, breathe out as you lower it down.

Breathe slowly and deeply

Breathe as slowly and as deeply as you can. If necessary, help evacuation by deep, slow breathing so that the abdomen moves in and out and the gut relaxes. Never hold your breath while passing stools.

Massage your tum

Gently but firmly massage your abdomen while sitting on the toilet. This encourages bowel emptying as well as improving general muscle strength and tone. I'd also recommend you try the massage that I described previously (see page 78). This helps to tone the valve between the small and the large intestine, which gets weakened by long-term constipation and straining.

Lift your arms

Try raising your arms to the sides, then above your head and back again in a slow, stretching movement. Repeat this several times. Or try rocking your upper body gently from side to side at the waist. Both these actions help to relax the lower part of the colon.

Give yourself time

Allow things to happen naturally.

Recommended reading

If you think your constipation might have an emotional cause, you might be interested in these two books: *Frontiers of Health* by Dr Christine Page and *The Healing Power of Illness* by Thorwald Dethlefsen and Rudiger Dahlke.

Reducing the risk of constipation

KATHRYN'S TOP TEN TIPS

1. Drink more fluid. Lack of liquid is a major contributor to constipation.

2. Eat more fibre. Page 271 tells you which type of fibre is best.

3. Eat more vegetables – and drink vegetable juice before meals.

4. Get moving. Regular cardiovascular activity also exercises your insides.

5. Massage your abdomen every day.

6. Make time for undisturbed visits to the toilet.

7. Don't ignore the urge. Go when you need to go.

8. Don't rely on laxatives.

9. Don't be a constipated personality.

10. See your GP if you are concerned about any changes in your bowel habit.

WWW

The National Digestive Diseases Information website, an organisation attached to the American National Institutes for Health, has an excellent section on constipation. Go to **www.niddk.nih.gov**

10.

What's Up?
Diarrhoea

> **Read this chapter if you have diarrhoea, or if you think you may have:**
>
> - Irritable bowel syndrome (IBS)
> - Candidiasis
> - Lactose intolerance
> - Food allergy
> - Intestinal parasites

This book is essentially about chronic (long-term) conditions that affect the gut, so I won't be looking in any great detail at the kind of infectious diarrhoea that medics call 'acute' (meaning of rapid onset with severe symptoms but of short duration), which we associate with food poisoning, traveller's tummy or viral stomach upset. I'm more interested here in those episodes of *non-infectious* inflammation or irritation that are so often a symptom of lactose intolerance, food allergy or parasites, or the troublesome and socially inhibiting nervous diarrhoea associated with irritable bowel syndrome. See also the sections that deal specifically with these conditions. This section of the book is intended to be read in conjunction with those main chapters.

Jargon buster

Diarrhoea is not a disease in its own right but a symptom of an underlying disorder. It is defined as 'the result of unduly rapid transit of bowel contents'. Simply put, the stools are loose and liquid and are passed more frequently than normal. Sometimes there is a sense of urgency and not always a great deal of spare time to make it to the bathroom.

Stress and anxiety diarrhoea

Everyone knows that emotional upset can bring on the runs. Modern jargon has now given us performance anxiety diarrhoea, or PAD, a new name for the old problem of abject fear having a far-reaching effect on our bowels. Nervous stress before an interview, panic prior to public speaking, the terror caused by a visit to the dentist or an imminent examination – all can bring on the dreaded diarrhoea.

For stress-busting ideas see page 304.

Constipated diarrhoea

You'll know already that a great many digestive disorders are made worse because of constipation, but did you know that diarrhoea can be a *symptom of* a constipated colon? Known simply as inadequate-contact diarrhoea, it happens when the walls of the colon become coated and clogged up with old faeces, and 'new' wastes are no longer able to come into direct contact with the colon wall. This means that the water content of the passing liquids and semi-liquids doesn't get absorbed, faeces aren't properly formed and it all rushes out as diarrhoea. However, this could still mean that you're constipated.

Dangers of dehydration

The greatest danger of any kind of diarrhoea, whatever its cause, comes from loss of fluid from the body and, with that fluid, depletion of essential minerals. What happens is this: when wastes move from the small to the large bowel, they're a sludgy liquid. Under normal circumstances, fibre in the stools soaks up water and shapes the faeces into firmish blobs. Any excess water is then reabsorbed into the bloodstream. If the bowel wall is irritated or there is infection or inflammation, the sludge from the small bowel rushes too quickly through the large bowel, with no time for fluid and electrolytes (mineral salts) to be reabsorbed. Instead, stools remain runny, carrying with them high levels of mineral salts. Result: the body becomes dehydrated. Attacks of short duration, of one or two days for example, don't usually cause any serious long-term problems, but repeated strikes can weaken the system and disturb mineral metabolism.

That's why, when someone has had an attack of diarrhoea, doctors talk in terms of 'replacing fluid and electrolytes'. The body is losing a lot of fluid with each urgent bowel movement, so the most important measure is to replace it. The easiest and quickest way to do this is to include a variety of fluids (see below).

Diarrhoea and surgery

Diarrhoea is often a side-effect of gastrointestinal surgery involving the removal of sections of the stomach, or small or large intestine.

Action plan for Diarrhoea

Your diet

Replace lost fluids and nutrients

Try the juices, tea and soup listed in the diagram opposite. In addition, you might try a mixture of tomato juice and sauerkraut; a leading Swiss naturopath tells me that this combination makes an excellent electrolyte replacement. Rehydration supplements, available at most pharmacies, 'sports' drinks and liquid vitamin and mineral drinks are also useful. Refresh from Biocare comes in sachets to mix with water or juice and contains vitamins with potassium, magnesium and fructooligosaccharides that have the additional benefit of encouraging friendly gut bacteria. Green foods such as sea plasma, spirulina, barley or chlorella help to boost nutrient levels and maintain electrolyte balance. Try Optimum Source Chlorella, Lifestream Spirulina or Pure Synergy from Xynergy

Apple juice
Blackberry juice
Blackberry tea
Carrot juice
Carrot soup
Cranberry juice
Mixed vegetable juice
Mixed vegetable soup
Vegetable broth

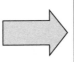

If possible, make your own fruit and vegetable juices and soups from organic ingredients. If this isn't an option, choose additive-free organic brands.

Also useful are:

Barley water
Chamomile tea
Japanese Miso*
Raspberry leaf tea
Slippery elm tea

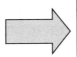

These drinks are usually available from health food stores.

*Miso is available in sachets from larger supermarkets and from some health food stores and delicatessens. Just mix with boiling water.

Health, Hawaiian Spirulina from The Naturopathic Health & Beauty Company or Sweet Wheat from Natural Woman. Stockist details are included in the Resource Directory (see page 323).

Note that orange juice is not recommended if you have diarrhoea. Although no one knows why, it seem to aggravate some ultra-sensitive systems.

Eat foods that might help

Small amounts of any of the following foods can help to calm and regulate erratic bowel movements:

Blueberries
Brown rice
Buttermilk
Cooked mashed vegetables
Grapefruit

Grated carrot
Mashed banana
Pears
Peeled and grated apple
Sheep's or goat's milk yoghurt

Carob powder has a long history of use as an anti-diarrhoea medicine, especially in Mediterranean countries. The effectiveness of this safe therapeutic is believed to be due to its high dietary fibre and polyphenol content. Polyphenols are natural chemicals that scientists believe have a protective effect on the body.

Udo's Choice Beyond Greens (Savant or Natural Woman) mixed into juice, oat porridge, yoghurt or soup provides nutritious green foods with dietary fibre, essential fats and healing herbs. It's the Rolls Royce of green food formulae and isn't cheap, but it would be my choice if I was recovering from a digestive upset and wasn't able to face ordinary meals.

> **Jargon buster**
>
> **Polyphenols** are nutrient components of plant materials, the most familiar being flavonoids, found in the pith, skin and bark of plants, and especially rich in dark-coloured berry fruits such as cherries, black grapes, blackberries, bilberries and cranberries, and in pine bark, green tea and grape seed extracts and, of course, carob.

Avoid drinking milk

If you're stricken regularly with diarrhoea but have no accompanying illness and cannot track down the cause, try giving up all cow's milk and related products for a week to see if there is any improvement. Lactose intolerance or inability to digest milk protein can both cause looseness of the bowel. Other symptoms of adverse reactions to milk may include floating stools, blood in the stools, constant tiredness, nausea after eating or iron-deficiency anaemia. See page 215 for more on milk.

Take care with vitamin and mineral supplements

Take care with vitamin and mineral supplements. A good basic daily supplement can be a valuable top-up to a healthy diet, especially where a gut disorder is linked to malabsorption or regular bouts of diarrhoea. However, certain nutrients – in particular magnesium and vitamin C – have a naturally relaxing effect on the bowel and could aggravate pre-existing diarrhoea if taken in too large amounts. Some cheap brands also contain ingredients that irritate the gut. I think it's best to choose really top-quality products that are specifically designed for people with poor absorption. I've found Viridian Multivitamins & Minerals and Biocare's Children's Multivitamins & Minerals (OK for adults, too) to be gentle on the stomach. Try Blackmores or Bioforce for Vitamin C.

Avoid artificial sweeteners

Some added sweeteners such as fructose or sorbitol can have a laxative effect and so are not recommended during the treatment of diarrhoea. Packaged fruit juices also seem to aggravate diarrhoea in some people.

Check your coffee intake

Coffee can be an irritant to some sufferers. It's usually recommended that coffee is avoided for several days in order to evaluate whether or not it's a culprit.

See if digestive enzymes will help

An inadequate supply of digestive enzymes from the pancreas can be a reason for loose stools. Digestive enzyme deficiency is a common problem that, except in very serious cases, usually goes undiagnosed. It's also aggravated by ageing and by many of the conditions discussed in this book. Try taking a month's course of top-quality digestive enzymes (one with lunch and one with your evening meal). If symptoms are markedly improved or eradicated, you'll know you've scored a hit. I would recommend Biocare Digestaid, Viridian Digestive Aid, Udo's Choice Digestive Enzyme Blend (available from Natural Woman or Savant), Solgar Vegetarian Digestive Aid or G&G Digestive Complex.

Note that digestive enzymes may not be suitable if you have gastritis, reflux or ulcers. Check with your doctor or nutrition practitioner first.

Check your fibre intake

The wrong kind of roughage can have an explosive effect on a sensitive gut, whereas the right kind can have an 'adaptogenic' effect, helping to ease constipation and, at the same time, calming a loose or irritable bowel. Page 271 tells you which kinds of fibre are best and which to avoid.

What else can you do?

Check for parasites

Diarrhoeal diseases due to parasites are still the leading cause of death throughout the world and, because of migration and increased travel worldwide and the consequent spread in parasitic infection, the numbers of people affected are also increasing in Western Europe and the United States. Parasites have been found to be linked to some cases of IBS diarrhoea. I suggest that you read Chapter 16 on intestinal parasites even if you don't think you're affected.

Take probiotics

Supplementation with *Lactobacillus acidophilus* is important in the treatment of all kinds of diarrhoea. A three-month course every twelve months makes good sense whatever your state of health and should be considered absolutely essential following antibiotics and/or bacterial infection. Important information on friendly bacteria and product recommendations are given in another section of this book (see page 294).

Treat allergies

Chronic diarrhoea can be a major symptom of food allergy, so one of the best ways of reducing the risk of attacks is to investigate and treat those allergies. As mentioned previously, one of the most common allergens is cow's milk, but other foods can be triggers, too. Chapter 12 contains more information.

Jargon buster

Lactobacillus is the Latin word used to describe lactic acid bacteria, one of the friendly bugs that helps to keep the gut healthy. Don't confuse the 'lacto' part of this word with the 'lacto' in lactose intolerance. There is no connection. Lactose intolerance (see page 215) is a condition in which the body is unable to digest lactose, the natural sugar content of milk.

Try these remedies

The following might help:

- Tormentil Complex (Bioforce) can be a useful treatment for infectious diarrhoea or antibiotic-related diarrhoea. It has a toning astringent action on the gut wall and also helps to expel parasites and bugs. **However, Tormentil would *not* be recommended in IBS-linked diarrhoea.**

- Avena sativa (oat juice) – also by Bioforce – contains compounds called iridoids that soothe the smooth muscle in the colon and calm it down. Avena also works on the central nervous system in general and therefore can help calm any nervous irritation that might be contributing to diarrhoea. Take five drops in about 2 centimetres (1 inch) of water once an hour until symptoms subside. Hold each sip in the mouth for thirty seconds before swallowing.

- A tablespoon of Silicea gel in a glass of water taken fifteen minutes before eating puts a protective lining over the digestive tract, helping to reduce inflammation. It also has a healing effect, as well as helping to expel bugs. This is a great product that usually works quite quickly. Some practitioners say that it is more effective than slippery elm. Silicea is available in most health food stores, or see Bioforce in the Resource Directory (see page 323).

- Molkosan lactic acid whey (Bioforce) not only knocks out unfriendly bacteria but also encourages friendly flora. Whey has an excellent record in treating intestinal complaints and flatulence, and should help to replace some of the minerals lost to diarrhoea. Dilute it in fruit juice or vegetable juice. See my extra notes on whey and lactose intolerance in the chapter on friendly flora (page 294).

Practise pelvic floor exercises

These help to strengthen the muscles around the rectal and anal area, reduce the risk of accidental leakage and 'wet wind', and help improve control in the case of urgent diarrhoea. See page 92 in the chapter on constipation for more information

See your doctor if:

- There is severe or blood-stained diarrhoea.

- Diarrhoea has persisted for longer than forty-eight hours and does not seem to be improving.

- The person affected is a child under ten years of age.

- You notice signs of dehydration such as strong body odour, sour breath, severe dryness of the mouth or lack of desire to empty the bladder.

- You see obvious dramatic weight loss.

If, for obvious reasons, you are unable to visit the surgery or health centre, ask for an urgent home visit. If a doctor is not available, ask to speak to the practice nurse or pharmacist.

Reducing the risks and side-effects of non-infectious diarrhoea

KATHRYN'S TOP TEN TIPS

1. Avoid cow's milk.

2. Drink lots of fluids.

3. Avoid wheat bran, bread and other wheat-based foods.

4. Include linseeds or psyllium in your daily diet.

5. Take regular courses of probiotic bacteria.

6. Get yourself checked for parasites.

7. Get tested for allergies.

8. Get tested for candidiasis.

9. Deal with stress and tension.

10. Keep non-drug anti-diarrhoea first-aid remedies to hand.

11.

What's Up?
Diverticulitis

❧ There should be an entire change in the dietary for a few days while taking opening medicine [and] the observance of a regular period of evacuating the bowels, which is most proper in the morning after breakfast. Skipping backwards, night and morning, is very useful. ❧

Cure For Constipation, *Enquire Within Upon Everything*, 1906

> **Read this chapter if you're suffering from:**
>
> * Diverticular disease
> * Constipation

What is it?

Diverticular disease is a condition where sections of the muscular wall of the large bowel weaken, become slack and form sac-like protrusions called diverticula. The actual condition is properly called diverticulosis; only when the diverticula become inflamed and/or infected does the condition become diverticulitis. Remember that any condition ending in 'itis' usually indicates some kind of inflammation.

What goes wrong?

Let's think back to the journey we took through the digestive system and, in particular, the large intestine. Wastes are pushed through this tube by a muscular action called peristalsis. If the muscles become weakened (through ageing, lack of exercise or lack of dietary fibre for example), they lose their elasticity, sag like old chins and form sacs or pouches. The 'pushability' of the colon is affected and, instead of 'moving right along', wastes collect and stagnate. This is diverticulosis.

If you think this all sounds uncomfortable, you'd be right. If you are a diverticulitis sufferer you'll already know how unpleasant the discomfort can be. It's an unpredictable condition with flare-ups of pain, nausea, diarrhoea, constipation and general malaise.

Jargon buster

Diverticula are the weak spots in the large intestine that bulge outwards into 'blind' pockets in the intestinal wall. Each singular pouch is called a diverticulum. More than one (i.e. plural pouches) are called diverticula or diverticulae.

Diverticulosis is the condition of having diverticula, so the two words can be taken to mean the same thing; in other words, those small pouches or sacs (diverticula) that form on the wall of the colon and get gunged up with waste products. Diverticulosis is sometimes referred to as 'diverticulitis without complications' because the early symptoms – constipation, bloating, abdominal cramps and occasional diarrhoea and discomfort in the lower left abdomen – are usually mild and may give no immediate cause for concern.

Diverticulitis is inflammation of the pouches and surrounding area. It's a complication of diverticulosis and occurs when particles of waste get caught up in one or more diverticula. When the inflamed diverticula become swollen and blocked with faeces, they are also swamped with bacteria that use up large amounts of B vitamins and disturb the balance of friendly gut flora. This can lead to inflammation and infection and, as the condition progresses, small perforations in the colon wall cause pain and tenderness in the lower left side of the abdomen. By far the most common symptom of diverticulitis is chronic constipation. Other symptoms include blood loss from the rectum, general abdominal discomfort, 'tummy upsets', and sometimes fever, nausea or vomiting, and general malaise. Where there are episodes of diarrhoea, the condition is often mistaken for – or confused with – irritable bowel syndrome.

Who is most at risk?

Diverticulitis is generally regarded as a disease of so-called civilised society because it's aggravated by rich, refined, low-fibre diets but rare in countries where the diet is unrefined. It's rare for the condition to develop before the age of forty but it does occur occasionally in younger people and is common in the elderly. In mid-life, the incidence increases dramatically and tends to match with age; for example, it's been suggested that 50 per cent of fifty-year-olds may be affected, 60 per cent of sixty-year-olds, and so on.

> ### Possible complications
> Most cases of diverticulitis are controlled by diet and medication. However, there can sometimes be complications. Severe bleeding may give rise to haemorrhage into the bowel. Seriously inflamed diverticula can perforate. Where perforated pouches don't heal, abscesses, pus and bacteria form outside the colon wall, leading to the life-threatening condition of peritonitis. In these cases, emergency surgery is usually required to drain the area and/or remove the affected section.

When to see your doctor

If you are suffering from any of the symptoms mentioned on page 106, I would strongly suggest that you ask your doctor for a check-up. While there is no evidence that either diverticulosis or diverticulitis increases the risk of colon cancer, some of the symptoms may be similar, especially where colon cancer affects the lower left side. Also, it is known that chronic constipation can be a precursor to cancerous changes, and constipation is one of the symptoms of diverticular disease. For these reasons, your doctor may recommend one or more investigative procedures to confirm the correct diagnosis and to rule out other conditions.

For more information on constipation see page 80. For more information on dietary fibre see page 271. See also *If You Do Nothing Else . . .* page 250.

In more detail

Diverticular disease is usually diagnosed by means of a barium X-ray, sigmoidoscopy or colonoscopy.

A **barium X-ray** can show up any intestinal obstruction in the large intestine. Because the inside of the bowel does not show up well on an X-ray, some preparation is required. Even a small amount of faeces caught up in the wall of the intestine can obscure information or confuse the picture. The night before the test, the patient is asked to drink a cleansing liquid to flush out the waste. Before the procedure the colon is filled with a chalky liquid that makes the whole area more visible on the X-ray. Although there may be a feeling of bloating when the barium fills the intestine, there is usually only mild discomfort, and after the procedure, stools may be a strange-looking white colour for a few days.

A **sigmoidoscopy** involves the use of a flexible tube called a sigmoidoscope. A light attached to the end of the tube allows the doctor to view the rectum and the lower part of the intestine, called the sigmoid colon.

A **colonoscopy** is similar in that it involves the insertion of a long, flexible tube with a light on the end of it, except that this tube is longer than a sigmoidoscope and enables the doctor to view the entire length of the colon.

None of these procedures could be classed as comfortable, but none is painful either. Prior to the sigmoidoscopy or colonoscopy you'll almost certainly be offered light sedation. During any of the tests there may be a sensation of wanting to empty the bowels, and you will probably feel gassy and bloated for a day or two afterwards.

Action plan for diverticulitis

For flare-ups

Try the following rescue remedies for diverticulitis flare-up:

- In acute situations, where there is a lot of discomfort and inflammation, symptoms may be helped by taking easily digested liquids or semi-solids just for a few days. Soups and juices are ideal for keeping nutrient and fluid intake high. Choose from carrot, lettuce, beetroot, apple and grape juices. Use organic fruits and vegetables wherever possible. Home-prepared juices are best but if you don't have a juicer, substitute bottled organic vegetable juices, which are available from health food stores. Make simple vegetable soups using carrot, broccoli, cabbage, celery and/or butternut squash. Chop the ingredients, cover with water and cook until tender. Blend to a smooth liquid, then reheat to serve.

● Green juices such as Spirulina, Chlorella, Barley, Oat and Wheat Grass are nutritious and easily digestible additions to your daily vegetable or fruit juice. Suggested brands are given on page 323.

● If these liquids are well tolerated, begin to add more solid foods. Good choices include raw grated apple, mashed banana, raw grated carrot, mashed papaya or mango, cooked mashed swede or sweet potato. Avoid ordinary potatoes and keep clear of fruit skins and any foods that contain hard seeds such as tomatoes, figs or cucumbers.

● When you begin to introduce high-fibre grains, stay away from wheat bran. Well-cooked brown rice is a gentle fibrous alternative.

● After the first week, start adding a teaspoon of ground linseeds to your daily vegetable juice. Use plain organic golden linseeds such as Linusit Gold. Simply put the seeds into the liquidiser first and grind them for a few seconds before blending the rest of the juice. Increase gradually to two teaspoons and then three teaspoons daily over the next few weeks. You probably won't need more than this if the rest of your diet is rich in fibre. Linseeds make an excellent regular fibre supplement to a healthy diet.

● Take a good-quality linseed or psyllium product every day. Chapter 22 has important information that you should read before increasing your fibre intake.

● Slippery elm powder makes a soothing 'tea', especially useful if taken an hour before bedtime.

● Blend a ripe banana and a teaspoon of Manuka honey into half a carton of sheep's or goat's milk yoghurt for a nourishing and soothing sweet treat.

- Once symptoms settle down, progress to a broad-based diet of fresh, unprocessed foods.

Your diet

Avoid potential 'irritants'

Avoid stuff such as orange juice, wheat bran, cow's milk and foods that are loaded with E numbers.

Choose oats instead of wheat cereal

Try oat-based muesli. It's kinder and more nourishing than 'string and sawdust' cereals. Or make smooth porridge with oat bran. Mix it with water, not milk, and sweeten with a teaspoon of New Zealand Comvita Manuka honey (available from health food stores, or see Resource Directory, page 323). I always recommend Manuka honey not just because it tastes great but because it has an anti-bacterial action and is gentle on the digestion. It's quite a bit more expensive than ordinary honey, but I think it's worth the extra cost.

Feast on dried fruits

Soaked dried fruits such as apricots, prunes and figs provide excellent fibre, plenty of nutrients and a sweet treat.

Find an alternative sweetener

Even if you suffer from a sweet tooth, it's really worth cutting back on sugar and avoiding artificial sweeteners. Manuka honey (see above) makes a useful alternative.

Cut the caffeine

Chemicals in coffee can also cause cramping.

It's OK to take some alcohol

Alcohol in small quantities has a relaxing effect on the colon so may actually be helpful in reducing spasms. How much? No more than one or two units (see page 51) per day. I don't need to tell you that drinking to excess has many detrimental effects on the body.

VERY IMPORTANT POINT

Seeds – good or bad?
You may have read that people with diverticular disease should avoid eating seeds and foods that contain seeds, such as tomatoes, grapes, strawberries and figs – or, indeed, linseeds, in case a seed might lodge in the diverticula pouches and cause blockage or inflammation. As is so often the case with nutritional advice, the experts disagree, and there is no scientific evidence to support or deny the theory.

The prestigious National Institutes for Health in America believe that there is no evidence for concern. Other equally highly regarded organisations say exactly the opposite. In a constipated colon disabled by diverticular disease, there seems little doubt that any kind of undigested food could aggravate bacterial overgrowth and increase the risk of inflammation and infection of the colon. But seeds are nutritious and many foods that contain them are the fibrous foods doctors recommend diverticulitis sufferers *should* eat. So perhaps the best plan would be to include seeds but, as I suggested earlier, to grind them first in a food processor. I would also urge you to take all other possible steps to make sure that everything you eat is chewed really thoroughly, and to keep fluid intake high.

Other top tips

Chew your food

Do this really thoroughly, and take time over meals.

Avoid cigarette smoke

Both yours and other peoples'. Nicotine doesn't only cramp your style; it cramps your colon by reducing blood supply to the intestines.

Take vitamin C

One or two grams of a low-acid or 'buffered' vitamin C before meals not only helps to improve regularity but may also reduce inflammation and the risk of infection. Avoid those large vitamin C tablets that you dissolve in water; they can be very acidic and may upset a sensitive digestion.

Try these remedies

To help to soothe inflammation and encourage healing of bowel tissue in diverticulitis, try Slippery Elm (Blackmores, Bio-Health, Solgar), taken with lots of water before meals. I've also had good reports about the use of Garlic supplements (Blackmores, Biocare) and Echinacea (KiwiHerb, Bioforce, Blackmores, Biocare) for helping the body to fight infection. (This is incidentally a great combination for colds, too).

Get moving

Exercise – walking, dancing, cycling, swimming, keep fit, yoga – improves blood flow to the colon and helps stimulate bowel activity.

Rub your tum

Follow the advice on abdominal massage described elsewhere (see page 78).

Try a castor oil pack

It may ease discomfort and draw toxins. This application works best if the person being treated is lying down. Apply cold-pressed castor oil directly to the skin of the area to be treated – for example, for the gall bladder and liver this will be over the right rib cage; for diverticulitis it will be on the lower left side of the abdomen. Cover with several layers of clean soft cloth (such as remnants from old cotton pillowcases or flannelette sheeting), cut to approximately 30 centimetres (12 inches) square. Over this, place some plastic wrap, such as a large polythene bag or clingfilm. Then place an old towel over the plastic wrap. Place a heat source (hot-water bottle or heating pad as warm as is comfortable) over the pack and leave it in place for an hour. At the end of this time, remove the layers, wipe off the excess oil and wash the skin gently with warm water in which you have dissolved a tablespoon of baking soda. Dry thoroughly and get dressed or put on night clothes so that you keep the area warm. Store the castor oil cloth in a polythene bag for the next use. For the best results, repeat the pack daily for three days. **Caution: don't take castor oil internally**.

What about bananas and rice?

A nutritional difference of opinion concerns bananas and rice, which some experts say should be avoided in diverticular disease because they are 'constipating'. Bananas and brown rice are, in fact, rich in dietary fibre and have the added advantage of being 'adaptogenic', meaning that they are good at settling diarrhoea as well as helping to ease constipation. It's worth pointing out that any kind of fibrous food has the potential to be 'constipating' if the diet doesn't contain enough fluid.

Most important of all

Up your fluid and fibre intake

An improved diet that includes an increased fluid and fibre intake can help to heal the intestinal walls, keep bowel movements regular and reduce the risk of further flare-ups. A gradual increase in fibre intake is the best way forwards. But be aware that however gently you introduce more fibre, there is a strong chance that you'll experience some bloating and flatulence. This is usually temporary and is a sign that your body is adjusting. Also bear in mind that drinking an adequate amount should be considered as important as any dietary changes (see page 289 for quantities).

Reducing the risk of diverticular disease

KATHRYN'S TOP TEN TIPS

1. Increase your fibre intake – but do it slowly. Learn the facts about fibre (see page 271).

2. Drink more water, and read Liquid News (see page 289).

3. Chew your food thoroughly.

4. Improve your digestion (see page 250).

5. Quit smoking if you do smoke.

6. Find a substitute for coffee.

7. Do more exercise, including Kegels (see page 92).

8. Enjoy alcohol in moderation.

9. Go when you have to go. Don't put it off.

10. See your doctor for a check-up to rule out other conditions.

WWW

Check out these websites for more information:
www.gutfeelings.com/diverticulitis.html
www.ukselfhelp.info/groupnadd.htm
www.niddh.nih.gov/health/digest/pubs/divert/divert.htm
www.fascrs.org/brochures/diverticular-disease.html

12.

What's Up?
Food Allergies

An amazing number of food allergies clear up completely when supposedly allergic individuals learn to eat their foods in digestible combinations. What they suffer from is not allergy . . . but indigestion.

Herbert M. Shelton, 1895–1985

Read this section if you think you're suffering from:

- Food allergies or sensitivities
- Unresolved weight problems
- Leaky gut syndrome
- Or if you think you're intolerant of, or sensitive to, a particular food

---

At some time or other, most of us suffer occasional nausea or stomach discomfort after a rich meal, or cave in to a craving we should really have avoided, or eat something and never know why it disagreed with us. We felt a bit liverish or queasy for a few hours but recovered and vowed not to do it again. These things happen; it was just a blip.

But what if you've reached the stage where you need to analyse every menu? To think about almost *everything* you eat, because you know from experience that certain foods, perhaps a list that seems to grow ever-longer, simply don't see eye to eye with your digestion anymore? Could they be food allergies?

Reactions to food are often dismissed as 'all in the mind' but being upset by 'something you ate' is nothing new, nor is it likely to be a figment of your imagination. Food allergies, often called food intolerance or sensitivities, have been implicated in a long list of different health problems and, some reports suggest, could be the cause of undiagnosed symptoms in vast numbers of the population.

Symptoms range from mildly uncomfortable to debilitating, the severity and type of response depending upon which part of the body has been 'attacked', by which particular 'alien' or allergen, and how that area of cells and tissues responds to the attack.

Symptoms and conditions

The symptoms and conditions linked to food allergy include:

All the symptoms of candidiasis
    (see page 65)
Anxiety
Arthritis
Asthma
Bloating
Bursitis
Coeliac disease
Dark patches under the eyes,
    known as 'panda eyes' or
    'allergic shiners'
Depression
Diarrhoea
Eczema
Enuresis (bed wetting)
Frequent urination
Palpitations
Fluid retention
Gastritis
Glue ear
Headaches
Hypoglycaemia

Insomnia
Intolerance to alcohol
Irritability
Irritable bowel syndrome
Itchy skin
Lower back pain
Migraine
Poor concentration
Poor digestion
Puffy eyes
Racing pulse
Recurrent ear infections
Rhinitis
Sensitivity to a range of foods
Severe fatigue
Sinusitis
Spaciness
Susceptibility to viruses and
    bacterial infections
Ulcerative colitis
Ulcers
Weight fluctuation

Causes and triggers

Likely causes or triggers of food allergy include:

Inadequate digestive enzymes
Inadequate levels of stomach acid
Inherited tendencies/family history of allergies
Insufficient natural antihistamines (possibly due to poor absorption or deficiencies of certain nutrients)
Intestinal parasites
Lactose intolerance
Leaky gut syndrome
The ulcer bug, *Helicobacter pylori*
Overgrowth of the yeast *Candida albicans*
Poor food combinations
Reduced liver or adrenal function
Rushed eating habits
Stomach upset, gastroenteritis or viral infection
Existing respiratory allergies
Excessive exposure to stress
Limited or restricted food choices
Reliance on processed, packaged foods

Before we go any further, let's make sure we understand what an allergic reaction is and what it does.

Jargon buster

An **allergic reaction** simply means an *altered* reaction, an abnormal response to a normal substance. It's nearly always to something that we find in our everyday surroundings, such as pet dander, pollen, dust or, in the situation we're looking at in this chapter, a food or component or contaminant in the food. We call the substance that causes the reaction an allergen or an antigen. This simply means any substance that, when it is introduced into the body, causes the formation of antibodies against it. Think of allergens as aliens.

It's generally accepted that most (although not all) food allergies, to a greater or lesser extent, involve the immune system, our internal 'army' that protects the body from viral and bacterial infections and from cancer. It's also called upon to deal with any invaders that the body doesn't recognise. When a food allergen enters the body, even though the food itself may be familiar and apparently harmless, alarm bells ring to warn the body that there is an alien in the camp and to call up its defences. Antibodies known as immunoglobulins (think of them as special forces) work with white blood cells to chase out the alien.

Jargon buster

Immunoglobulins are antibodies, protein substances manufactured within the body that are designed to 'lock on' to any alien invader to neutralize it, slow it down or exterminate it.

The two groups of allergies

The two main goups of allergies are *true* (also called *fixed* or *classic*) allergies and *cyclical/cumulative* allergies. To confuse us all even more, as mentioned above allergies may also be referred to as food intolerance or food sensitivity. Depending upon your source of information, these terms are used interchangeably to mean the *same* thing or, alternatively, they refer to *completely different* kinds of allergic response. I've tried to disentangle the terminology not only for your benefit, but for mine too!

True allergies

These are sometimes referred to as fixed allergies, classic allergies, or food anaphylaxis, and they are thankfully relatively rare, accounting for anything between 1 and 3 per cent of cases. Symptoms are usually severe and immediate. If you're unfortunate enough to belong to this group, the chances are that you'll already know it. This kind of allergic reaction is often genetic in origin and therefore a lifelong hazard. Some of the most common antigens include peanuts, seafood, nuts and eggs, but it's possible to be allergic to absolutely anything. It makes no difference how often or how infrequently the sufferer comes into contact with the antigen; it will always be a problem. The tiniest amount of a substance can throw the body's immune system into panic and chaos, causing large quantities of powerful inflammatory chemicals known as leukotrienes and histamine to be released.

Bloods vessels dilate and fluids are lost from the circulation, creating a dramatic drop in blood pressure. The throat and tongue swell up. Toxins are released, sending the bronchioles (breathing tubes) into spasm, and causing a severe asthma-like reaction and suffocation. The resulting shock, known as anaphylaxis, can occur within seconds, minutes or a few hours of coming into contact with the offending food.

Sufferers usually need to carry emergency supplies of adrenalin (called epinephrene in the United States) which, when injected, counteracts the effects of the histamine by opening up the airways and recovering the breathing. Even a moment's hesitation can be fatal. If you suffer from this form of allergy, do take extra care when buying packaged foods or when eating out because a problem food may be hidden among otherwise harmless ingredients.

Snippets

The drugs we know as antihistamines are prescribed to cancel out the histamine reaction. However, they are usually only used to ease the symptoms of respiratory allergies and not food reactions.

Cyclical allergies

These are also referred to as cumulative allergies, and they develop – as the name suggests – by repetitive and continued eating of the same offending food, and account for the majority of cases. It's widely accepted that excessive and repeated consumption of a limited number of foods or food ingredients is one of the major reasons behind the huge increase in food allergies. However, many of the people who suffer from this type of allergy are unaware that their symptoms are actually being 'self-propelled' by familiar everyday foods, such as wheat or dairy products. One reason for this is because any reaction can be delayed for hours or even days, making it extremely difficult to isolate or identify the little devil that caused the trouble.

But this doesn't mean that food allergies are a new health problem. Hippocrates, the ancient Greek physician and founding father of medicine, observed that milk could cause stomach upsets and skin irritation.

He clearly understood cyclical allergies, writing that it can be 'the commencement of serious disease when [someone takes] twice a day the same food which they have been in the custom of taking once'. In other words, a small quantity of a particular food may cause no problems but double the amount of that food could trigger symptoms.

In cyclical allergy, if the offending food is avoided for several weeks or months, it may be the case that it can be reintroduced and enjoyed without any adverse reactions, as long as it isn't included too frequently. The diet that is usually employed to overcome cyclical allergy is known as a Rotation Diet, or Rotary Diversified Diet.

Food Intolerance

This is a term that is sometimes taken to mean food allergy, but it also refers to someone who has either lost – or never had – the ability to digest a particular food because of an enzyme deficiency; most usually the term is used to describe lactose intolerance where there is a deficiency of the enzyme lactase, needed to digest milk sugar. The immune system is not involved in milk intolerance. However, cow's milk that is fed consistently into a body that has no enzymes to digest it could, over time, become an allergen and cause an immune system alert by the very fact that the milk remains undigested and therefore a potential trigger for other conditions such as leaky gut syndrome.

For more information on lactose intolerance see page 215.

Intolerance to gluten, which is a component of some grain crops, and predominant in wheat, does involve immune system reaction. There's more on gluten in the leaky gut syndrome chapter (see page 222).

Food intolerance may also be linked to a psychological trigger such as being forced to eat a particular food in childhood; the memory of an unhappy event associated with a food can resurface in later life to resemble an allergic reaction.

Food sensitivity

This is a relatively new term that is being used to describe a reaction to any food that causes digestive grief, bloats you up, makes you feel nauseous or leaves you exhausted and spaced out. Food sensitivities are often the result of leaky gut syndrome. Reactions are linked primarily to the digestive system and may also be responsible for other symptoms, including weight problems, joint pain and skin flare-ups. Although not everyone agrees, some allergy specialists are tuning in to the idea that the immune system may be involved in food sensitivity, just as it is in true food allergy (see page 118), although to a far less severe extent and without endangering life. It certainly seems to follow that most food sensitivity is down to low stomach acid or deficiency of digestive enzymes – in other words, to poor digestion (see below).

Other reasons for food reactions

Could it be down to a defective digestion?

It's natural from most of what I've said so far to assume that whatever ails you is a food allergy. But have you ever considered the possiblity that your reaction might be brought on by an *inability to digest*? I'm certainly not the first nutritionist to observe that some of the symptoms of suspected food reactions are akin to those of sub-standard digestion, and that a great many cases of so-called allergy clear up completely when the gut is healed and the digestion is improved.

American Dr Herbert Shelton, who spent much of his career investigating the different ways in which food could affect the digestive system, observed that an amazing number of food sensitivities cleared up completely when people who thought they were allergic began to eat their meals in what he termed 'digestible combinations'. No, nothing to do with edible underwear, but everything to do with eating foods that fit the natural pattern of digestion, rather than loading the plate with foods that are bound to fight, not just each other but the digestive system, too. Dr Shelton's view that starches are not digested properly if eaten at the same time as proteins did not find favour with many of his medical colleagues. However, his extensive research, and that carried out by other practitioners before and since, seems to confirm that food combining does indeed improve the quality of digestion.

I'm not suggesting that this scenario applies to everyone with allergies. Clearly, allergic reactions are extremely common and very genuine. However, my own experience with patients shows either definite progress or sometimes complete clearing of 'allergic' symptoms when the digestion is improved.

The system can't cope

It's seems highly likely that the human body simply can't handle the massive change in dietary habits that has occurred over the past half century. Our digestive system, which is still working as it was some 40,000 years ago, is suddenly faced with a highly processed diet consisting of unnaturally produced, hybridised or otherwise modified or altered substances that it isn't used to; 'plastic' foods preserved and denatured to the point where we have difficulty recognising the original ingredients.

System overload

Some researchers and allergy specialists believe that the lower the immunity and the higher the exposure to potential allergens, the greater is the likelihood of allergic reactions. Known as the Total Load Concept or System Overload Theory, this simply means that someone is much more likely to react – or overreact – to an allergen (whether it be food, chemical or airborne inhalant) if their immune system is underfunctioning and therefore unable to deal with the invader.

If a person is properly nourished, eating a varied diet, getting plenty of rest, not smoking or using 'social' drugs, drinking alcohol only in moderation and not excessively or repeatedly stressed, then it follows that their immune system is likely to be strong enough to withstand ingress by those 'aliens' we talked about earlier. However, if your body is under a lot of negative stress, you get snatched sleep and rely on packeted meals, or have an otherwise restricted diet, with regularly missed meals, or if you are exposed to cigarette smoke or other heavy pollution (for example if you work in a polluted area or drive in heavy traffic) this is creating just the right terrain for allergies to take hold. And if you already suffer reactions to pollen, house-dust mites, animal fur and so on, you could be a more likely candidate for food reactions.

New chemicals

Compounding the problem further is the fact that the vast majority of commercially produced 'convenience' food is loaded with a range of relatively new chemicals in the form of artificial preservatives, colourings, flavourings, stabilisers and emulsifiers, to which neither the body in general, nor the immune system in particular, has had time to adapt.

Processed foods

Despite our rapid, almost frightening, 'progress' in science, technology and communication, and huge improvements in our living conditions, perhaps we haven't made such good progress when it comes to our food supply. Our supermarkets may appear to be bursting with variety, but take a closer look. The diversity of fresh produce that dominated the hunter-gatherer/Stone Age diet has been replaced with a more limited and not-nearly-so-natural supply of foods based on hybridised wheat and corn, factory-farmed meat, pasteurised and mass-produced milk, highly refined sugar and manufactured fat, and laced with an astonishing array of man-made chemicals including artificial additives and crop-spray residues that have been around for only a few years. This has happened within a space of time that isn't long enough for our bodies to even begin to adapt – a mere nanosecond in evolutionary biology.

Over-acid system

A diet that is short on vegetables and fruits can cause the bloodstream to be too acid. There is some clinical evidence to suggest that, by increasing intake of alkaline-forming fresh vegetables and fruits, the number of adverse reactions to food is reduced. This may be because the nutrients in those foods are valuable for boosting immunity or perhaps because most fruits and vegetables are generally easier for the body to digest than heavy-duty acid-forming meat, grains and processed foods. Or perhaps it's simply the case that, as we include more fruits and vegetables, we naturally eat less of the foods likely to cause reaction.

Leaky gut syndrome (LGS)

This is a condition where the wall of the small intestine 'springs a leak' and allows substances through into the bloodstream that shouldn't be there. The result in an increase in allergic reactions. For more information on leaky gut syndrome and its link to food allergies, turn to page 222.

Could food allergies cause weight problems?

It's common to meet people who complain of putting on weight even though they know, they absolutely know for sure, that their activity levels are about the same as they were when they were slimmer and they haven't consumed any extra calories. Obesity experts will usually say that this isn't possible, that it's easy to eat more without realising it or that any extra weight gained is bound to be caused by overeating and/or underexercising.

If you've been struggling to lose weight but, in spite of extra exercise, a calorie-controlled diet and huge helpings of willpower, you've made little or no progress, you might be interested in trying a different tack.

The idea that food reaction could actually be causing a weight problem is still controversial. Just as contentious is the concept that poor digestion may also contribute to someone being overweight. But work with patients and feedback from them suggests pretty strongly that some cases of overweight respond extremely well not just to improving the diet but to improving the digestion, too. There could also be a link between food allergies and that uncomfortable bloat we associate with fluid retention. When food allergens irritate and inflame the gut, the body responds by trying to 'flood out' the irritants and, in the process, accumulates extra fluid which, in turn, can lead to unwanted 'water weight' or fluid retention. In addition, some of the chemicals that are released during this process not only slow up the metabolism, reducing our ability to burn fat, but they may also make us want to eat more; as a result, of course, we put on more weight.

Action plan for food allergies

There are many simple changes to diet and lifestyle that can help to reduce the risk of food reactions but, before trying anything else, I'd give priority to *three main moves*. The suggestions I'm making here are those that I've collected over ten years of clinic work and from feedback from patients. I hope they help you too.

If what you have is a cyclical or cumulative food allergy, then one of the most effective ways to treat the problem is to avoid the food that causes the reaction. Sometimes this is easy. At other times, deciding which foods (if any) are the real troublemakers can be a thorny problem.

It's perfectly possible to have specific allergies to absolutely anything, but equally important to realise that what causes a reaction in one person may not do so in another: a classic case of one person's meat being another person's allergen.

Stage 1 – better your digestion

Sometimes the symptoms that seem like an allergy are, as I've explained above, more likely to be connected to poor digestion. It is for this reason that my first recommendation is to do whatever you can to improve the way your body digests its food. This may be one of the most important moves you can make towards improving your health. Pages 251–270 are therefore essential reading.

Stage 2 – eliminate the *big three* problem food groups

Wheat-based foods

These foods, and in particular wheat cereals and bread, are a common cause of indigestion, bloating, irritable bowel, mental 'fogginess' and general lethargy. Feeling *tired all the time* is a frequent complaint from people who eat a lot of bread. Rye bread, rye crackers, oat biscuits and rice cakes are nourishing alternatives to the breakfast toast or the lunchtime sandwich. Oatmeal, oatbran, rice, rye, quinoa or millet couscous (avoid wheat couscous) are cereal options. It's worth knowing that spelt and kamut (although still wheat) are often well tolerated even by those who cannot cope with regular pasta. Wheat-sensitive pasta lovers could try rice pasta. (If you give up wheat and wheat-containing foods, you'll also be cutting your intake of gluten. There's more on gluten in the chapter on leaky gut syndrome, see page 222.)

Cow's milk

This is equally hard for many people to digest. A small amount in a cup of tea does not usually cause much mayhem, but in larger amounts – by the glass or poured on to cereal – it can cause acidity, mucus and sticky stools. Try oat milk, rice milk or organic soya milk instead. And go for sheep's or goat's milk cheeses and yoghurts instead of cow's milk equivalents.

Food additives

Check labels and avoid artificial food additives including E102 tartrazine colouring, E110 sunset yellow colouring, E220-E227 sulphite preservatives, E250 sodium nitrite preservative and colour fixative, and E621 monosodium glutamate flavour enhancer. Avoid all artificial sweeteners including sorbitol, saccharin and aspartame.

All the items that I've mentioned in Stage 2 cause symptoms in so many people that it really is worth trying to manage without them. You could get lucky and, like others that I've met, feel much better and not need to take your sleuthing any further.

If you're still searching for clues, then move to . . .

Stage 3 – Consider a course of probiotics and digestive enzymes

Invest in top-quality products and take them every day. The probiotics will help to repopulate the healthy bacteria in your colon. The digestive enzymes will take the strain off your digestive system, giving it a rest and ensuring that you properly digest your meals. As we age, our bodies may produce less stomach acid or fewer digestive enzymes and, as a natural consequence, food won't be broken down or assimilated as efficiently as it used to be. Good combinations to look out for? Biocare Bio-Acidophilus with Biocare Digestaid capsules, Blackmores Digestive Aid and their Acidophilus/Bifidus, Solgar Advanced Acidophilus and Solgar Digestive Aid, Udo's Choice Digestive Aid with Super 5 or Higher Nature Probiogest with their Supergest Digestive Enzymes.

If you feel better at the end of the month and can afford to do so, I would suggest taking the probiotics and digestive enzymes for a further two months. This is not a cheap option, but I'd always consider quality supplements a priority ahead of, say, buying clothes, cosmetics or a new mobile phone. Never forget that your health is your wealth.

Further investigation

If you're not improving as a result of the suggestions I've already made above, then you'll need to get down to some more detailed investigations.

Check for other troublemakers

Even if you don't have an allergy problem, the items on this list are probably best consumed in only the smallest quantities:

Sugar	Orange juice
Eggs and chicken that aren't organic	Yeast
Coffee and cola	Corn
Shellfish	Gluten
Peanuts	Tap water

Beware of related foods

Foods that belong to the same species or botanical family may, for some people, cause similar reaactions because they have the same protein or chemical structure. That's why someone allergic to cow's milk may also react to beef. If you have a problem with prawns, you might be well advised to steer clear of other shellfish, too. Some foods may cause reactions not because they are directly related but because they contain the same additives. Simple testing that avoids certain 'food families' – just for a few days – can be a reliable way of routing out the troublemakers. *The Wright Diet* by Celia Wright contains an excellent chapter on food tests that you can do safely at home. If you cannot find it in a bookshop or library, contact Higher Nature. Their address is in the Resource Directory (see page 323). *The Encyclopaedia of Natural Medicine* by Michael Murray and Joseph Pizzorno also has useful 'food family' tables.

Play around with combinations

If you still get no result in your search for what ails you, it's really worthwhile playing around with food combinations. I've known quite a few food-sensitive souls who, although they didn't react to any of the above individual groups, found that the mix was the problem. For example, one patient was upset by cheese only if she ate it with bread. A cheese salad caused her no discomfort, but a cheese sandwich was 'painful'. Another lady found that tomatoes only aggravated her digestion (and her arthritic joints) if she ate them cooked *and* ate the skins. Raw and peeled tomatoes were absolutely fine. A third patient who came to see me for advice about reducing cholesterol, weight and dyspepsia, discovered that a scrambled egg breakfast was well digested and so, too, was toast (he had no wheat or egg sensitivity), but if he ate them together as scrambled eggs on toast, the resulting digestive discomfort stayed with him all day. There's more on simple food combining on page 283.

Did you know?

'A series of papers (was) published in the Lancet and elsewhere a few years back on the subject of Adulteration. These brought about a parliamentary inquiry which concluded that nearly everything we ate and drank was adulterated – in many cases with ingredients very prejudicial to human health. The result was the passing of an Act of Parliament for the purpose of putting a stop to this wholesale adulteration by making it a criminal offence . . . called the Sale of Foods and Drugs Act. "No person shall mix, colour, stain or powder any article of food with any ingredient or material, so as to render the article injurious to health, with the intent that the same may be sold in that state, and no person shall sell such article under a penalty not exceeding £50." '

Think this quote was written recently? No, it comes from *Enquire Within Upon Everything*, published in 1906 by Madgwick, Houlston and Co. Ltd.

Nothing changes very much!

Go organic

Sometimes it can be the food additives or other chemical residues and not the food itself that are causing the problem. I've known people react to ordinary chocolate but be unaffected by organic chocolate! I can tolerate a small amount of organic cow's milk but get catarrh and indigestion if I drink the smallest quantity of the non-organic version. Where people react to barn- and battery-raised poultry and eggs but not to organic free-range produce, this may suggest intolerance not of the foods but of drug residues, artificial colours, hormones or other chemicals in the mass-produced versions. It's probably worth emphasising here that 'organic' and 'free-range' do not mean the same thing. Hens, for example, may be free-range in that they are allowed to roam outside but may still be fed on non-organic foodstuffs. When choosing poultry and eggs, free-range is likely to be better than battery or barn-raised fowl, but organic free-range will be better still.

Did you know?

Chlorinated water can cause quite severe indigestion. I've known several people who've spent months trying to isolate the particular food that they thought was upsetting their digestion only to discover, eventually, that it was the chlorine in their tap water.

The answer? Filter it.

Watch out for your favourite foods

It's worth noting that people often say they feel better when they concentrate on eating only their 'favourite' foods. Ironically, however, foods that figure prominently in the diet, that is they are eaten every day or several times a day, are often found to be the culprits. It makes working out what to eat and what to give up an extremely difficult task. If you give up or cut back on your favourites and feel worse for a while, that may indicate withdrawal symptoms. The complicated nature of trying to sort out food allergies and intolerances makes practitioner support absolutely vital.

Don't restrict your diet

So many different foods are potential triggers that you may think it's best to give up almost everything and see what happens. Take care. In the same way that a limited diet can create food allergies in the first place, restricting food choices still further could cause your system to become sensitive to the few foods that remain. There is also a big risk of serious malnourishment because you're just not eating a wide enough range of nutrients. Short-term exclusion diets can be helpful in some cases but it is *neither necessary nor safe* to follow them for long periods of time. Indeed, a few over-zealous allergy therapists have been criticised – probably with justification – for removing too many potential allergens from the diet for too long and not properly monitoring nutritional status and progress of symptoms. I cannot stress too strongly the need for vigilance when dealing with food allergies or intolerances.

Are you eating really fresh food?

Always check the use-by date on everything you buy and make sure it's consumed well within that date. Foods that readily attract mould should be viewed with caution (even if you are not allergic to the foods themselves) since moulds are well-known allergy triggers. So make sure that you use only the freshest items. I always remember the advice given at a health lecture by nutrition expert Geoffrey Cannon that we should eat food that goes bad *before it goes bad!* How wise. It is generally the case that the most nourishing foods are those that will, under normal circumstances, deteriorate the quickest; that is fresh, whole, unadulterated produce. Highly processed and refined foods with added preservatives are not likely to contain the same level of nourishment as their fresh equivalents.

Foods that can attract mould may therefore aggravate allergic reactions. Such foods include:

Alcoholic beverages
Bread and other baked goods that contain yeast
Canned and cartoned juices
Canned foods, especially tomato products
Cheeses
Cold cuts of meat
Cooked rice
Dried fruits
Herbs, chilli and curry
Mayonnaise, salad cream, foods containing vinegar
Milk, cream and yoghurt
Mushrooms
Peanuts
Pickles and relishes
Sauerkraut
Smoked fish
Smoked, preserved meats
Soy sauce
Stock cubes and yeast extracts

This doesn't necessarily mean that it's wise to give up all these foods. Just be aware how important it is to eat everything in a really fresh condition.

Consider other conditions

Following on from what I said in the previous paragraph, if you have an ongoing problem with food reactions, you need to look into the likelihood that there could be another underlying illness such as candidiasis or leaky gut syndrome. Check out the chapters on these two possibles and see if the symptoms match your profile.

Check for the ulcer bug

Helicobacter pylori has been implicated by one study as a possible cause of food allergies. If you're not improving, despite all your best efforts, see your doctor and ask to be checked for *H. pylori*.

Be wary but sensible

If you think a particular food is really troublesome, remove it from the diet for the short term and follow this Action Plan (see page 124), reintroducing the suspect after a gap of three months. You may find it causes you no problem at all because by that time you're digesting all foods more efficiently. What it all comes down to in the end is this: if your health ain't so great and you're not improving, despite medical or other treatments, investigate the possibility that certain foods might be a problem – but avoid a food only if you are absolutely certain that it is affecting you detrimentally. *Don't dodge something just because you've heard or read that it causes allergic reactions in someone else.*

Deal with stress

It's well known that, when the body is under continued stress, allergic reactions can be more severe. One theory for this is that allergic individuals have a shortage of the particular white blood cells that are needed to make antibodies. It's also known that, under stress, levels of IgA (for definition, see page 296) are much reduced. IgA works out of the mucous membrane, where it puts up a barricade to keep out foreign substances. It's believed that people who suffer from allergies, in particular those of the cyclical type, have unusually low levels of this particular immunoglobulin antibody, anyway. By succumbing to the effects of negative stress, the situation is made worse.

Browse your local health food store

Look for organic, dairy-free, wheat-free, gluten-free foods. Pester your local supermarket to stock the specialist food products that you need. Orgran, Village Bakery, Everfresh, Trufree, Doves Farm, Goodness Direct, Kallo and Lyme Regis Foods are just a few of the labels to look out for. They all have websites; try looking for them using a search engine such as Google or Yahoo.

Testing for allergies

I have deliberately not dealt with testing in this chapter. This is a specialist area that requires practitioner guidance and is something that you should consider if your efforts so far have not resolved your symptoms. I'd strongly suggest you find an experienced and qualified clinical ecologist or allergist who has a proven track record in treating food reactions and can carry out a range of recognised tests. If possible, arrange to be referred by your GP.

Need more help?

Food Matters At The Inside Story – a quarterly newsletter containing useful articles, recipes, new product news, latest findings and an extensive list of self-help and support groups, valuable to anyone suffering from food allergies or food intolerances. Very highly recommended. Contact *Food Matters At The Inside Story*, Berrydale House, 5 Lawn Road, London NW3 2XS, enclosing a large stamped addressed envelope for subscription details, or see website below.

Action Against Allergy is an excellent resource and may be able to help you if you're looking for a practitioner in your local area who can help treat allergies. Contact them at P.O. Box 278, Twickenham, Middlesex TW1 4QQ. See also website below.

Recommended reading

Jonathan Brostoff & Linda Gamlin, *Food Allergy and Intolerance*, Bloomsbury.
Lynda Brown, *New Shoppers Guide to Organic Food*, Fourth Dimension.

Rita Greer, *Gluten-Free Cooking*, Thorsons.
—— *Wheat, Milk & Egg-Free Cooking for Health*, Thorsons.
—— *Wheat-Free Cooking – Practical Help for the Home Cook*, Souvenir Press.
Ellen Rothera, *Encyclopaedia of Allergy and Environmental Illness*, David & Charles.
Celia Wright, *The Wright Diet*, Clearlight Books, available from Higher Nature (see page 323).
Food Adulteration and How To Beat It (London Food Commission).

Reducing the risk of allergies

KATHRYN'S TOP TEN TIPS

1. Take care not to restrict your diet: eat as wide a variety of foods as possible.

2. Cut right back on the problem foods that I've talked about in this chapter and make a real effort to introduce some of the alternatives I've suggested.

3. Increase your intake of fresh vegetables and salad foods.

4. Reduce your use of household chemicals and use biodegradable products around the home.

5. Avoid packaged meals and takeaways: prepare meals from scratch so that you know what goes into them.

6. Regularly repopulate your friendly gut flora (see probiotics, page 294).

7. Filter your tap water.

8. Go organic whenever and wherever possible.

9. Understand the basics of food combining (see page 283).

10. **Make improving your digestion an absolute priority** (see page 251).

www.inside-story.com
www.foodsmatter.com
www.allergyfoundation.com
www.allergy.co.uk
www.actionagainstallergy.co.uk
www.niaid.nih.gov/factsheets/food.htm
www.kidshealth.org, then search food allergies.
www.medlineplus.gov, search food allergies.
www.stamp-collection.co.uk has information on their fab range of
    wheat-free, dairy-free foods, recipes and useful links to other sites.
www.soilassociation.org
www.chemicalbodyburden.org
Find the Food Standards Agency website page at
archive.food.gov.uk/committees/cot/cot000727.htm
(Note: Don't put www at the beginning of this address.)

13.

What's Up?
Gallstones

Gallstones can be round, oval or faceted, grains of sand or pieces of fine gravel, or they may develop as just one large painful pea, mammoth marble or gigantic golf ball. A single piece might completely fill the gall bladder. Size obviously matters because quite a lot of people who have surgery for gallstones will be given their 'trophy' to put on display.

How do we get them?

Gallstones form when there is an imbalance in the constituents of bile, which is manufactured by the liver and stored in the gall bladder.

Jargon buster

Bile is a liquid that is used to help digest fats in the diet and also enables us to absorb fat-soluble vitamins A, D, E and K. Bile is made in the liver and then stored in the gall bladder until it's needed. When we eat a meal that contains fat, the gall bladder is triggered to contract, pushing bile though a tube – unsurprisingly called the bile duct – which is then directed into the small intestine, where it helps with digestion. Bile is made up mostly of water, cholesterol, lecithin, bile salts and a substance called bilirubin, which gives the bile (and also our stools) a brownish/yellow tinge. If the bile gets too concentrated (that is, overloaded with too many bile salts, too much cholesterol or excess bilirubin) it can solidify into the pieces of hard material that we know as gallstones.

> ## Jargon buster
>
> The **gall bladder** is an expandable, pear-shaped pouch tucked just under-neath the liver on the right-hand side of the body, underneath the lungs behind the rib cage.

How do gallstones happen?

Instead of being able to flow through the bile duct, gallstones get stuck either in the gall bladder or, if they've managed to move along a bit, they might get wedged in the cystic duct (gall bladder exit) or common bile duct which joins it to the small intestine.

There are four types of gallstone. Which type you get depends to a large extent on where and how the imbalances occurred, and on the ratio of the bile ingredients and its solubility. Put simply, soluble bile flows freely, clogged bile doesn't. If the cholesterol increases or the bile salts or the lecithin decrease, the bile thickens and gets gooey. It's at this stage that the tiniest particles in the bile begin to attract cholesterol around them and form into gravel and then, ultimately, into stones. It's estimated that, once this process begins, stones can increase in size by around 2.5 millimetres a year.

Pure cholesterol stones are formed – it's easy to guess – from hardened cholesterol. They're most likely to occur if, for some reason, the gall blad-der doesn't empty as it should, and if the balance of ingredients in the bile is disturbed (that is, if there's too much cholesterol and not enough bile salts). These stones are common in the affluent Western hemisphere and less so in underdeveloped nations.

Pure pigment stones form from bilirubin, which is why they are brown. They're most often associated with biliary tract infections, parasitic infections, cirrhosis of the liver or sickle cell anaemia. Still relatively rare in the West, this type tends to be more common in Asian countries, where there is a higher frequency of parasitic infections of the liver and gall bladder. There is also some evidence that they may be linked to sun exposure.

Mixed stones are made up of cholesterol, pigment, calcium and bile salts. In affluent countries, these tend to be the most common type of gall-stone.

Mineral stones are made up predominantly of calcium, but may also contain silicon or aluminium oxides.

Which comes first?

If you're wondering which comes first, the gall-bladder disease or the gallstones, in most cases the order is something like this:

- As a result of dietary or other factors, bile thickens up and slows down.
- The gall bladder doesn't empty as it should.
- Bile solidifies into stones.
- Tubes become blocked.
- The gall bladder distends and becomes inflamed.
- Emptying is further inhibited.
- Result: gall-bladder disease, actually called cholecystitis.
- Gallstones are found in nearly all people who are suffering from gall-bladder inflammation.

In more detail . . .

All the tubes and ducts associated with storing and transporting bile and digestive enzymes from the liver, gall bladder and pancreas to the small intestine are known collectively as the biliary system. That's why, when we feel a bit off-colour, we use the term 'bilious' or 'liverish'.

The hepatic duct takes bile out of the liver; the cystic duct carries bile to and from the gall bladder; and the common bile duct transports bile from the cystic and hepatic ducts to the small intestine. Bile that solidifies and gets trapped in any these ducts can cause inflammation in the gall bladder, in the ducts themselves or, occasionally, in the liver. If a gallstone blocks the opening to the pancreatic duct, digestive enzymes – which should be on their way to the small intestine – get trapped in the pancreas and cause an extremely painful condition known as gallstone pancreatitis. As you can imagine, if any of these passageways remain blocked for any length of time, the outcome isn't just excruciating – it could cause permanent damage to the liver or pancreas.

Likely symptoms?

It's perfectly possible to have gallstones and yet have no symptoms at all. You may never be troubled by them and never know you have them unless stones show up in tests that are carried out for some other reason. People who have these 'silent stones' are said to be asymptomatic (without symptoms). When symptoms do occur, we usually refer to the episode as a 'gallstone attack' simply because they come on suddenly when the gall-bladder wall becomes inflamed or because stones have moved out of the gall bladder and blocked one of the ducts. Most commonly, attacks occur after a rich, fatty meal or during the night. Other symptoms can include:

Abdominal bloating
Belching
Colic
Constipation
Fullness
Gas
Headaches
Indigestion
Irritability
Knife-like pain in the upper right quadrant
Nausea or vomiting
Pain between the shoulder blades
Pain in the abdomen
Pain under the right shoulder
Quick sharp temper
Recurring intolerance of fatty foods
Severe discomfort after a meal that contains fat

What puts you at risk?

Crash dieting	So don't do it. There's plenty of evidence that very low-calorie weight-loss programmes are a risk factor for gallstones. What happens is that, as the body metabolises fat during rapid weight loss, the amount of cholesterol in bile is increased, making the formation of stones more likely.
Fasting	Fasting has a similar effect to crash dieting. The sudden reduction in calories slows down gall-bladder contractions and causes the bile to become over concentrated with cholesterol. So don't do it unless you are very familiar with the procedure and have medical support.
Low-fibre, high-fat, high-sugar diets	Consider this kind of diet to be 'superfood' for gallstones. Refined carbohydrates, sugar and the wrong kind of fats all serve to upset the solubility of bile and decrease bile flow.
Food allergies	Sensitivity to certain foods is believed to aggravate gallstones. Eggs, pork, onions, poultry, milk, coffee, citrus fruits and juices, corn, legumes (pulses) and nuts have been identified as possible triggers. The first three on this list seem to be the most problematic. But this doesn't necessarily mean that everyone with gallstones is allergic to any or all of these foods.
Diabetes	People with diabetes are likely to have higher levels of blood fats (known as triglycerides) than people who don't have the condition and this increases the risk of gallstones. It's also possible that insulin might play a role here, by stimulating the body to produce more cholesterol.
Being female	Unkindly, it used to be said that the typical gallstone personality was fair, fat, flatulent, female and forty, an alliteration familiar to medical students the world over. Although obviously sexist and discriminatory, it's still true that risk factors are higher for women of this age group who are overweight and suffering from constipation and poor digestion. But other criteria no longer fit. The age gap is now wider: women between twenty and sixty years of age are between two and four times as likely to develop gallstones as men. There may also be a genetic link. Native American women over the age of thirty – seven out of every ten, in fact – are at high risk for gallstones. Yet only 10 per cent of black women in the same age group are affected.

Hormonal problems	Excess oestrogen from pregnancy, the contraceptive pill or HRT appears to increase cholesterol levels in bile and slow down gall-bladder movement, both of which can lead to gall stones.
Eating meat	Vegetarians appear to be at lower risk of gallstones than meat eaters.
Crohn's disease and cystic fibrosis	In these two conditions, the secretion of bile is affected and reabsorption of bile acids is impaired, increasing the risk of gallstones.
Being a sun worshipper	So far this suggestion has been put forward by only one piece of research. However, the figures are alarming. In a study of 206 white-skinned subjects, those who sunbathed for long periods had twice the risk of gallstones as those who did not sunbathe.
Being older	As in the majority of diseases, ageing plays a role. Those over the age of sixty are more likely to develop gallstones than younger people.
Being overweight	Obesity is a major risk factor for gallstones, most probably because the fat factor slows down gall bladder emptying as well as reducing the amount of bile salts in bile, resulting in more cholesterol. You don't need to be seriously overweight. Being moderately heavier still increases your risk. It's also a fact that the heavier you are, the less well controlled are your insulin levels which, in turn, can unbalance your cholesterol.
Taking cholesterol-lowering drugs	I'm afraid it's contrary but true. Drugs that lower cholesterol levels in blood actually increase the amount of cholesterol secreted in bile which, of course, can increase the risk for gall stones.
Being inactive	Lack of exercise encourages decreased bile secretion and a greater likelihood of bile statis (incomplete emptying of bile from the gall bladder and bile solidifying into stones).
Being stressed	Stress is a negative factor in any illness.

VERY IMPORTANT POINT

See your doctor *without delay* if you are suffering from any of these symptoms:

- Any kind of pain anywhere in the abdomen or diaphragm that comes on rapidly and lasts between twenty minutes and several hours.
- Persistent or severe abdominal pain during the night.
- Chills or feverishness.
- Clay-coloured stools.
- Sweating.
- Yellowish colouring of the skin, nails or whites of the eyes.

Urgent and accurate diagnosis is vital. It's easy to confuse the pain of gallstones with the pain of appendicitis, diverticulitis, heart attack, hepatitis, hiatus hernia, irritable bowel syndrome, pancreatitis and ulcers.

If your doctor thinks you have a gallstone, he or she will probably send you for an ultrasound examination. The test is completely painless and is over in a few minutes.

If gallstones are found and they are causing you a lot of pain, the likeliest course of action will be surgery. Most gall-bladder operations are done with a tiny instrument called a laparoscope. This makes a much smaller incision than regular surgery, resulting in a shorter stay in hospital.

Medication to dissolve stones is available and may be offered, especially if surgery is not an option. However, it can take an extremely long time (months or years) to work.

What happens if the gall bladder is removed?

Most doctors will tell you that the gall bladder is not considered an essential organ so losing it is not usually a problem. When the gall bladder has gone, bile flows out of the liver through the hepatic ducts into the common bile duct and goes directly into the small intestine. All it means is that the storage facility for bile has been removed. The only likely side-effect of this redirection is that bile tends to flow more frequently into the small intestine and, as a result, can cause diarrhoea in some people. Because there's just a chance that this could elevate blood cholesterol, your doctor might suggest that you have more regular cholesterol checks. It's probable you'll be told that you should be a bit more careful about what you eat but that a change of diet might not be necessary.

Having said all that, many naturopathic practitioners believe that removing the gall bladder is a drastic step that does nothing to correct the reasons behind the gallstones that formed in the first place. Perhaps it's like having heart surgery to bypass blocked arteries but doing nothing after the operation to try to prevent the new tubes around the heart from clogging up? Bile is there for a purpose; it's important not only in fat digestion but also for the absorption of fat-soluble nutrients. It's also a key player in the detoxification department. If it's possible to improve the quality of the bile and in so doing restore the health of the gall bladder so that bile functions as nature intended, then I think it's worth looking at dietary improvements first and surgery as a last resort.

Action plan for gallstones

A typical diet of white bread, biscuits, coffee, sweet, sugary foods, bacon and eggs, rich sauces, takeaway meals, saturated and hydrogenated fats and general processed junk food is believed to be the best way to encourage gallstones – and, of course, a whole range of other unwelcome diseases. Dietary therapy is, therefore, aimed first at eliminating any foods that seem to aggravate symptoms. If you choose this route, I would very strongly suggest that you do so only with the guidance of a health practitioner. Seek a consultation with a qualified nutritionist or naturopath who is familiar with the condition and with the natural methods of treating it.

The dietary information included in this chapter is designed to help you reduce your risk of gallstones occurring or recurring. It is not presented as an alternative to surgery or medical advice.

Your diet

Cut back on coffee

Whether it's pukka percolated, filtered, instant or decaffeinated, coffee can aggravate symptoms by causing the gall bladder to contract. Studies also show that the same reaction occurs in healthy coffee drinkers who have no history of gall-bladder problems!

Avoid processed fats and oils

Swap them for sensible amounts of organic cold-pressed nut and seed oils. See my note on olive oil at the end of this chapter.

Avoid mayonnaise and salad dressings

Instead, make your dressings with a little extra-virgin olive oil, fresh lemon juice, garlic juice and organic honey. Or mix olive oil with organic cider vinegar.

Cut that fat

You should especially try to avoid processed fats, hydrogenated margarine-type spreads, butter, cheese, cream and meat. And check labels for any foods that are made with hydrogenated fats or oils.

Say no to sugar

Do you have to add sugar to beverages? Why not use quality organic honey instead? Try to cut back on sweets, cakes and biscuits, chocolate and any foods that are made with sugar. White or brown sugar can raise blood fats (see my note on cholesterol at the end of this chapter) and, research suggests, seems likely to increase the risk of gallstone formation.

Give eggs the heave-ho

Sure, they're a nutritious food, but they do seem to irritate already irritable gall bladders. This may be due to their cholesterol content or to the fact that they are also, sadly, a common allergen. Whatever the case, eggs are best avoided if you have the slightest sniff of gall-bladder trouble.

Leave off the legumes

Pulses – peas, beans and lentils – are almost always suggested as a healthy food because of their fibre content. But, for gallstone sufferers, there is a suspicion that they may not be helpful. During studies of Native Americans, Chilean and Pima Indians, all of whom have high rates of gallstones, it was noted that they had correspondingly high intakes of legumes. The connection could be genetic and nothing at all to do with the beans but, until research confirms one way or the other, beans may be best avoided or eaten only occasionally.

Drink more liquid

Filter water and try to drink six to eight glasses per day. Extra fluid helps to prevent gallstone formation. More information of the importance of fluid intake is included in Chapter 24.

Increase your fluid intake throughout the day. Include apple or pineapple juice (freshly squeezed where possible), chamomile tea, dandelion 'coffee', Bambu coffee substitute, Miso or vegetable soup.

Up your dietary fibre

I know I keep saying this throughout the book but it is so very important. If you haven't been there already, check out Chapter 22. Increasing dietary fibre has been found to lower cholesterol levels and may influence the bile acids that are involved in lowering cholesterol and dissolving stones.

Eat more fish?

I haven't been able to find any negative research showing that fish is bad for bile or that it gunges up the gall bladder. It makes a nutritious alternative to fattier proteins like cheese, eggs and meat. If oily fish doesn't agree with you, why not try white fish such as whiting, haddock, hake or plaice? There are also some interesting animal studies, by the way, showing that fish-oil supplementation may reduce the risk of stone formation.

Go veggie

Vegetarian diets are believed to be protective against gallstone formation. Since meat is shown to aggravate gall-bladder inflammation, it could make really good sense to swap some meat meals for vegetarian alternatives.

Give yourself five

Make a real effort to introduce at least two pieces of fresh fruit each day, plus a salad and two or three servings of vegetables. Not only are these foods low in fat, they are packed with vitamins, minerals and dietary fibre and should help to lower cholesterol. Fresh fruits and vegetables are also good providers of vitamin C, a nutrient that is strongly believed to be beneficial in beating and preventing gallstones.

Lose weight slowly

If you decide to lose some weight, begin slowly and carefully. Crash dieting can increase your risk.

Do everything you can to improve your digestion

Do everything you can to improve your digestion. Good digestion improves the transit time of food through the gut. Slow movement of food increases the risk of gallstones. Introduce as many as possible of the hints in the chapter If You Do Nothing Else . . . (see page 250).

Check out the section on constipation (see pages 80–95), and get those bowels moving. When constipation is resolved, gallstone risk appears to be much reduced.

What else can you do?

Don't smoke

There, I've said it again.

Try lecithin supplements

Lecithin has many beneficial actions. In particular, it has an emulsifying effect on blood fats and helps maintain normal cholesterol levels, and so may reduce the risk of gallstones. It is available in granules from your health food store (check the label and make sure it's not genetically modified soya). Or try Biocare's Lecithin Capsules. The Resource Directory on page 323 has contact information.

Snippets

The word lecithin is derived from the Greek word meaning egg yolk because that's where the substance was first isolated. Nowadays, most good lecithin supplements are derived from non-GMO soya.

Consider digestive enzymes

Lipase is a digestive enzyme that helps with the digestion of – guess what? – fats and oils. When you don't digest fat properly, chances are you won't be absorbing some important nutrients, in particular vitamins A, D and E. And you could be putting your gall bladder under pressure. One capsule of lipase daily (or a broad-spectrum enzyme complex that has lipase, and protein and starch digesters as well) with your main meal could help to take the strain off the gall bladder and pancreas and reduce the discomfort caused by eating. Again, I would recommend Biocare for Lipozyme Fat Digesting Enzyme or their Digestaid Enzyme Complex, Digestive Aid from Viridian, or Solgar Vegetarian Digestive Aid.

Take vitamin C

Vitamin C taken as 2,000 mg daily has been shown to have a beneficial effect on the composition of bile and to reduce stone formation. One of my favourite brands is Blackmores Bio-C because it's so gentle on the digestion.

What about peppermint oil capsules?

These may help to dissolve existing gallstones. Leading naturopaths Michael Murray and Joseph Pizzorno suggest a dosage of one or two capsules of 0.2 ml three times daily with meals. But do make sure you use enteric-coated capsules. Ordinary gelatine capsules without enteric coating can dissolve quickly in the stomach and may cause gastric discomfort.

Herbal help

Cholagogues are herbs that encourage the gall bladder to contract; herbs known as choleretics help to stimulate bile production and increase the liquid flow of bile. Both actions could be of value in reducing the risk of gallstones. Any herb that has a beneficial action on the liver is also likely to be of value to the health of the gall bladder.

- Milk thistle (*Silybum marianum*) is potentially one of the most useful herbs because it has rejuvenating action on the liver. It's also a potent antioxidant and helps increase the production of new liver cells. It is available in capsules but also as Milk Thistle tea with ginger and dandelion root from Biocare.

- Globe artichoke (*Cynara scolymus*) is known to help gall-bladder function, possibly because it regulates bile production. Arkopharma and Lichtwer Pharma both have a good Cyanara product.

- Turmeric (*Curcuma longa*) has a revitalising effect on the liver.

Note that most herbs are not suitable during pregnancy or during an acute gall-bladder attack.

VERY IMPORTANT POINT

If you're interested in using herbs, don't self-medicate. Seek professional help. If you are attempting to treat a gall-bladder condition using either herbal or homoeopathic medicine, I would caution against self-medication and strongly recommend that you consult a medical herbalist or qualified homoeopath.

Ask about acupuncture

This can be the most amazing therapy for pain control and may be especially helpful in reducing the spasm associated with gall-bladder pain. 'Needling' also helps to improve the flow of bile and enhance proper liver and gall-bladder function. Ask your doctor about a referral to a qualified acupuncturist.

Use a castor oil compress

The compress that I mentioned in the section on diverticulitis (see page 105) can also be very soothing for gallstone pain.

Wish away your gallstones

Try using guided imagery to dissolve your gallstones. It's important to be rested and relaxed, so first follow the progressive relaxation exercise (see page 316). Then sit quietly and picture your gallstones dissolving like melting butter in a warm frying pan. Once they've all melted to liquid, take some pieces of kitchen paper and wipe around the inside of the pan, soaking up the oil. Make sure the pan is thoroughly cleaned, then throw the buttery paper into the rubbish bin. Not only are you picturing dissolving your gallstones, but you are also throwing them away. Repeat this exercise as often as you can.

Reducing the risk of gallstones

KATHRYN'S TOP TEN TIPS

1. Cut right back on saturated and hydrogenated fats.

2. Don't get constipated.

3. Check your fibre intake.

4. Swap meat meals for vegetarian and fish ones.

5. Avoid eggs.

6. Drink more water.

7. Eat more fresh vegetables.

8. Lose weight if you need to but don't crash diet.

9. Improve your digestion.

10. Don't smoke.

Author's notes

About blood cholesterol

It seems that there is no correlation between the level of cholesterol in the blood and the amount of cholesterol in bile. And even though some research suggests that increasing HDL (the good cholesterol) and decreasing LDL (the sticky, not-so-nice cholesterol) might improve bile consistency, further studies don't reach the same conclusions. However, there does appear to be a link between an increase in blood fats (triglycerides) and stickier bile. Following my Top Ten Tips (see opposite) should go a long way towards improving the levels of blood fats and of the 'healthy' HDL cholesterol.

About the gall-bladder flush

You may have heard about 'gallstone-dissolving' diets, usually based on extra-virgin olive oil and fresh fruit juices such as grapefruit, lemon, apple and black cherry, and vegetable juices including raw beetroot juice, carrot and watercress. I have met several people who are convinced that the 'olive oil flush' worked for them, causing them to pass huge gallstones. However, the experts, as is so often the case, are divided.

Some say that these are not, after all, excreted gallstones but soft lumps of minerals, and that the stone still remains where it was – in the gall bladder. There is concern that, while olive oil and juices can be very good cleansing therapy for the liver, they do not help those with gallstones because the oil can cause the gall bladder to contract, increasing the risk of stones blocking the bile duct and requiring immediate life-saving surgery. And although not yet observed in humans, there are animal studies showing that olive oil can increase the content of cholesterol in the gall bladder itself, thereby making cholesterol stones more likely.

This view is not supported by legendary naturopathic Doctor H.C.A. Vogel, nor by my own nutrition tutors. Following conversations with other nutritionally oriented practitioners and patient feedback, my view would be that small amounts of cold-pressed extra-virgin olive oil and other cold-pressed nut and seed oils can be a useful symptom-free alternative to butter and processed oils. Perhaps the answer is to avoid any kind of drastic diet, and to avoid saturated fats and fatty foods, but to include small quantities of good-quality oils as part of a normal diet.

If you want to know more about gall-bladder tests and how they're done, or need information about surgical and non-surgical treatment, these websites are well worth a visit.
www.gallstones.upmc.com/Diagnosis.htm
www.mydyspepsia/infotesting.htm
www.tummyhealth.com

14.

What's Up?
Haemorrhoids/Piles

Read this chapter if you think you might have:

- Haemorrhoids
- Constipation

A haemorrhoid, or pile, is a varicose vein in or around the anus or lower rectum that is swollen and inflamed. In other words, it's a normal vein that has become abnormally enlarged or dilated, usually as a result of some kind of pressure on the blood vessels. The word haemorrhoid (or hemorrhoid in some countries), comes from the Greek *haimorrhoia*, meaning 'flow of blood'.

What causes them?

Most of our veins have valves inside them to make sure that blood only flows in one direction, to the heart. The veins around the anal area drain into larger veins on their way to the liver and back to the heart.

Unfortunately, this part of the venous system has no valves and so the whole weight of the blood being transported is able to 'bear down' on the veins lower in the system, restricting the flow of blood, putting them under pressure and causing them to stretch. If a vein is under strain and it has no valves, blood back-flows into balloon-like pockets, producing varicose veins or haemorrhoids. Anything that brings a stress or force to bear on the pelvic and abdominal area, such as constipation, can increase the risk of haemorrhoids.

Who is at risk?

Here is yet another ailment that is often cited as a 'modern' complaint, being blamed, at least in part, on the highly processed 'Western' diet. It's true that haemorrhoids are rare in countries where unrefined whole grains are a major ingredient in the diet, and widespread in societies that eat rich, refined and processed foods. But although haemorrhoids are a common disorder, they are also mentioned in some pretty old manuscripts. For example, one fifteenth-century text refers to a good medicine 'for the pylys and the emerawdys', which I take to be either the ancient spellings for piles and haemorrhoids or the names of old Welsh villages.

It's believed that at least half the population of affluent countries has haemorrhoids by the age of fifty. Men and women are affected equally. However, incidence also increases with age, as muscle tone slackens and bowels tend to become increasingly constipated.

Signs and symptoms

The most common symptoms of haemorrhoids are:

- Burning, pain and general discomfort
- Difficult bowel movements
- Feeling of fullness in the rectum
- Feeling of lumps or swellings in or around the anal area
- Mucus in the stools
- Red blood on the loo paper
- Sensation of incomplete evacuation

- Itching can be a symptom, although anal/rectal irritation is more likely to be caused by allergic reactions to the texture or chemicals in toilet paper, excessive use of harsh soaps or bubble bath, parasitic infections, *Candida albicans* overgrowth or food allergies.

If you have an external haemorrhoid you may notice:

- A painful swelling, hard lump or the sensation of 'extra skin' around the anus.

- If skin tags become inflamed, there may be a feeling of pressure in the back passage. Large veins can be very uncomfortable, especially during bowel movements. Skin tags and enlarged veins can also make it hard to clean the anal area, which in turn can encourage itching, burning, irritation and soreness. Excessive straining, scratching or cleaning may cause even more irritation and lead to a vicious cycle of symptoms.

- If you don't feel able to ask your partner or carer to examine your anal area, you can see quite a lot by sitting in a squat position using a mirror and a good light. However, the simplest and safest way to check for any problems – and to put your mind at rest – is to see your medical practitioner or practice nurse.

If you have an internal haemorrhoid, you may notice:

- Bright red streaks of blood on the surface of the stools, on the toilet paper or in the toilet bowl.

- As you're passing stools, the bulging of the haemorrhoid in the anal canal can give you an uncomfortable feeling of fullness. It's been likened to the sensation of not having completely evacuated your bowel. And a protruding haemorrhoid can feel like a flappy bit of skin sticking out around the anus, not unlike an external haemorrhoid. See how difficult it can be to differentiate between the two types? If it doesn't recede on its own, try pushing it gently back with a finger.

- Larger haemorrhoids may swell as they are squeezed by the muscles (anal sphincter) that control the opening and closing of the anus. They may also secrete mucus, causing mild skin irritation and itching. Proper hygiene helps to reduce the risk of discomfort but take care to treat the area gently. At their worst, large internal haemorrhoids stick out of the anus all the time. These large swellings can become extremely painful if they are rubbed, scratched or otherwise irritated during over-zealous cleaning.

153

What causes and aggravates them?

Anything that puts pressure on the blood supply to the abdominal and pelvic areas could bring on or aggravate haemorrhoids, including:

Being overweight	Overeating
Chronic constipation	Undue straining
Lack of dietary fibre	

Other possible triggers include:

Anal intercourse	Laxative abuse
Carrying heavy loads	Poor abdominal tone
Chronic stress	Poor circulation
Crossing the legs	Poor posture
Family history	Tight clothing
Lack of exercise	Toxic colon

Constipation, haemorrhoids and varicose veins are also commonly associated with pregnancy. The combination of hormonal changes, increased blood flow to the pelvis and the obvious pressure of the foetus in the abdomen causes the blood vessels in the anal area to enlarge. Those same blood vessels are, of course, put under severe strain during childbirth. However, haemorrhoids during pregnancy are nearly always only a temporary problem.

Treatment – an overview

Although many people have haemorrhoids, not everyone is aware of them because not everyone will have symptoms. Haemorrhoids are not usually dangerous or life-threatening. It's also comforting to know that, in all but the most severe cases, simple medical treatment together with dietary improvements are enough to eradicate symptoms. However – and it's a big however – once the small blood vessels have been stretched and dilated and scar tissue has formed, removing local damage can be difficult.

Treatment is therefore aimed at preventing a recurrence rather than curing the condition.

In more detail . . .

For most people, a pile is a pile is a haemorrhoid, and all they want to know how to relieve the discomfort and reduce the risk of recurrence. But, in case you're interested, here's more detail.

External haemorrhoids may be thrombotic (when a blood vessel ruptures and forms a clot), or cutaneous (made up of fibrous connective tissue covered by outer skin). What usually happens is that a vein is put under pressure and bursts, causing blood to 'pool' under the skin and create a painful thrombosed haemorrhoid. You'll know if you have one. A severely blood-clotted haemorrhoid can be excruciating, so bad that you can't walk or sit down with any degree of comfort. Over time, the blood clot is replaced by a lump of tissue and, although the discomfort may remain, the pain recedes.

Internal haemorrhoids, as I've explained already, occur above the anorectal line but can feel pretty much the same as an external haemorrhoid to the uninitiated, which is why an examination and diagnosis can be essential. Mostly, internal ones are not painful. But sometimes, an internal haemorrhoid can enlarge to the point where gravity takes hold and it descends (prolapses) below the anal sphincter. This pushy behaviour seems to give the internal variety a bit more clout in medical terms – important and complicated enough for haemorrhoids in this category to be graded, like peas, according to their size.

I sometimes wish I didn't have that weird sort of mind that has to wonder what job title they give to someone who grades piles for a living, although I have heard it said that a bum doctor who starts out at the bottom and stays there is called a proctologist. However, I digress:

Grade I Means that the vein bulges or swells during bowel movements but doesn't protrude from the body.

Grade II Describes a vein that bulges during bowel movements and actually comes out of the anus but goes back in by itself.

Grade III Indicates that the vein comes out during bowel movements and stays out, requiring finger pressure to push it back in.

Grade IV Refers to a vein that sticks out all the time and is resistant to being pushed back.

Having **mixed or internal/external haemorrhoids** simply means that someone is suffering from both kinds of piles at the same time.

Did you know?

The patron saint of piles is the sixth-century Irish Saint Fiacre. Whether he suffered or not isn't documented.

Jargon buster

It's easy to confuse the symptoms of haemorrhoids with **anal fissures**, the skin tags that result from a tear in the wall of the anus. Both fissures and haemorrhoids can cause bleeding and severe pain, especially on defaecation; fissures also become infected. Several other back passage problems, including abscesses, irritation and itching (pruritus ani), also have similar symptoms and can be mistaken for haemorrhoids.

Snippets

It is recorded that piles were a trait of the family Bonaparte and that Napoleon suffered abysmally with constipation and piles throughout the Battle of Waterloo!

Seeing your doctor

See your doctor in any of the following events:

- If you notice any kind of bleeding that has occurred for no apparent reason and is not associated with emptying your bowels.

- If your stools are narrower than usual – in other words in thin sausage strips rather than rounded fatter ones.

- If you notice any kind of lump near the anus.

- If an existing haemorrhoid gets much bigger or bleeds.

- If pain or swelling due to existing haemorrhoids worsens.

- If you have any seepage of mucus or any unidentifiable material from the anus.

- If stools appear much darker in colour than usual or have the consistency of spent coffee grounds.

- If you feel the need to empty your bowels but are unable to do so or if you have not had a bowel movement for more than four days.

Note: in rare cases, the opening and closing of the anus may cut off the blood supply to the swollen veins. This causes tissues inside the rectum to die and emergency surgery is required to prevent serious damage.

Checking out your symptoms

These recommendations are not intended to alarm you. I include them simply because it's important for your doctor to be able to rule out other, more serious, diseases that might require urgent attention.

As I've said previously, please don't be embarrassed at asking your doctor or practice nurse to examine you. To a medical practitioner, examining someone's backside is no different from checking their pulse or looking down their throat. It's all in a day's work. Most importantly, your doctor will be pleased to be able to put your mind at rest.

When you go for your consultation, the doctor will probably examine the anus and rectum and check for any swollen or protruding blood vessels that indicate haemorrhoids. This will almost certainly involve a digital rectal examination with a gloved, lubricated finger and/or instruments that allow the doctor to either to see any internal haemorrhoids or to have a good look inside the rectum. For a more detailed examination, you might be referred to a specialist for a sigmoidoscopy (examining the rectum and lower part of the intestine called the sigmoid colon) or a colonoscopy to view the entire colon.

If haemorrhoids are confirmed, your doctor is likely to prescribe one or more items to help relieve your symptoms. These may include:

- Lubricant cream or suppositories to help ease difficult bowel movements.

- Stool softeners to help reduce straining and prevent hard stools.

- Laxatives to 'bulk up' the stools and help prevent constipation.

- Rectal preparations to relieve itching, discomfort and pain.

Nutritional treatment, consisting of an improved diet, the right kind of fibre and correct fluid intake, together with vitamin and herbal supplements known for their blood-vessel strengthening and skin-healing properties – especially if used in conjunction with medical treatment – can be very successful and may avoid the need for painful surgery.

Action plan for haemorrhoids

Your diet

If you already suffer from haemorrhoids, making a few simple changes to your daily routine can help you to manage the symptoms and feel much more comfortable. It's estimated that at least half of all sufferers feel better when they do nothing more than improve their diet.

VERY IMPORTANT POINT
Drink more fluid. Check out pages 289–293 for the Liquid News.

Take in more roughage

Include more of the following in your diet: fresh vegetables and fruits, and whole grains such as oats, rye and brown rice. Soaked prunes, figs and apricots make a delicious high-fibre sweet treat. For more important facts about fibre, be guided by the special section on page 271.

Don't rely on bran alone

Bran is a good treatment for relieving the symptoms of haemorrhoids but shouldn't be considered a single or complete answer. Remember that it's better to eat a wide-ranging, wholefood diet rich in vegetables, fruits and unrefined cereals than it is to stay with a low- fibre, high-fat, high-sugar diet and simply try to remedy the fibre issue by adding bran or fibre supplements.

Helpful hint

Linseeds are an excellent fibre to use if you're recovering from surgery for piles. Not only are they rich in nutritious oils and fabulous fibre, but they're also blessed with mucilagous (slippery) and demulcent (soothing) qualities that ease the passage of wastes through the wounded area. Bowel movements in the weeks immediately following this operation, known as a haemorrhoidectomy, have been likened to passing broken glass. If this is happening to you, can I suggest that, at least until you have recovered, you try a product called Linoforce from Bioforce. Read the information on Linoforce in the section on dietary fibre (see page 278).

Eliminate refined and low-nutrient foods

These include sugar, caffeine and alcohol.

Limit dairy products

Keep dairy products to a minimum. Cow's milk may seem like a nutritious option but, unfortunately, it does seem to increase mucus production and to 'glue up' the digestion, slowing down the passage of wastes through the system for some people.

Take in the right minerals

Include plenty of foods rich in calcium and magnesium. The list on page 87 tells you which foods contain which mineral.

Eat the right kind of fats and oils

Cut back on saturates and hydrogenated spreads. Give up ordinary cooking oils. Introduce extra-virgin olive oil, fresh oily fish, seeds and, unless you're allergic, eat more nuts. Walnuts, Brazil nuts and almonds are especially nutritious. Include two or three teaspoons of cold-pressed oil in your diet every day. The box on page 251 has more information on this.

Eat berries and grapes

Include lots of blueberries, bilberries, blackberries, cranberries, cherries, black grapes and raspberries in your diet. They're rich in antioxidant nutrients known as flavonoids which are needed to strengthen blood capillaries; some particularly special flavonoids are called proanthocyanidins. Don't be put off by the name. It's just a Greek word meaning the dark colourings found in plants and, especially, the blues, reds and purples of berry fruits.

Consider daily supplements

- **A regular vitamin and mineral supplement** that has the right balance of nutrients should help to promote healing and assist in relaxing the rectal and anal muscles. Check that yours contains vitamins A, all the Bs, C and E, and the minerals zinc and magnesium. There's no need to take masses of different pills. Just invest in a multi-tablet or capsule (plus extra vitamin C, below) and buy the best that you can afford. Good choices? I'd recommend one a day of the Earth Source Multi-Nutrients from Solgar or Viridian's Multivitamin & Mineral Formula. If swallowing pills isn't your thing, boost your diet with one of the nutritious powders now available. Try Viridian Organic Green Food Blend mixed into juices or smoothies, or one of the 'green' foods mentioned on page 244.

- **Vitamin C** is essential for healthy connective tissue and healing. What isn't always well known is that C-rich foods as well as vitamin C supplements have a naturally laxative effect; a particular boon if you're struggling with the pain of piles or recovering from haemorrhoid surgery. So eat lots of fresh fruits and vegetables and take a daily vitamin C capsule or tablet. Good-quality brands include Biocare, Blackmores, Solgar, Bioforce and Viridian.

- **Glucosamine sulphate and chondroitin sulphate** are naturally occurring compounds found in the structure of cartilage and blood vessels. The names may be familiar to you if you use these natural medicines to ease the pain of arthritis. There is evidence to suggest that these two substances, especially if used with flavonoids such as blueberry, bilberry, rutin and hesperidin, may help prevent haemorrhoids by strengthening the blood vessels and improving blood flow.

Limit your alcohol intake

There's nothing wrong with having a drink; it can be enjoyable and help you to relax. However, more than one unit per day can lead to dehydration, which encourages constipation and so, you know by now, increases the risk of piles.

Be sensible about salt

Too much sodium increases the risk of fluid retention, which in turn can cause swelling and aggravate the pressure on the veins.

> **VERY IMPORTANT POINT**
> The greatest danger of salt overload isn't from sprinkling salt used at the table but from packaged foods. Bread, dried soups, canned foods, breakfast cereals, biscuits, stock cubes, ready meals and, of course, salty snacks, are a few of the most serious culprits. Just four slices of bread, two rashers of bacon and a couple of sausages exceed the daily recommended intake of 6 grams.

What else can you do?

Don't be constipated

The best way to prevent haemorrhoids is to prevent constipation and, consequently, avoid straining. Softer stools pass more easily than harder ones, thus decreasing pressure.

Improve your eating environment

Give your digestion a chance. Make your eating environment relaxed. Eat smaller, more frequent meals if you are used to eating large ones. Chew your food thoroughly. And *never* eat standing up. You're likely to eat too quickly and to have poor posture; neither is good for your digestion.

Get into toilet training

Practise the toilet training I recommended previously (see page 91). Make every effort to maintain healthy bowel habits and go to the bathroom as soon as you have the urge to move your bowels. Relax, don't rush or strain. Just let things happen naturally. Take a lightweight book and read a few pages – this takes your mind off the task in hand and helps to stop you from feeling pressurised. Take a couple of heavier books to use as footrests (see page 93). However, don't hang around in there for ages; sitting for too long can put additional pressure on the haemorrhoidal veins. If nothing happens, try again later.

Go for short walks

Avoid prolonged sitting and/or standing at work or during leisure time. Take frequent breaks and go for regular short walks.

Snippets

According to medical textbook opinion, the belief that standing or sitting in one position for long periods causes piles is nothing more than an old wives' tale. Well, as an expert old wife, I'd like to expand on this assertion because I think it gives the impression that these static activities are actually OK. While it's true that sitting or standing, especially on cold surfaces, is extremely unlikely to be the *trigger* for anyone's haemorrhoids, the *pressure* of sitting – and more especially standing – in one place for long periods of time does seem to make the symptoms of existing haemorrhoids – and varicose veins – much worse. Squatting, stretching, reaching and climbing (especially ladders and steps) should also be undertaken with caution.

Kick the laxative habit

Long-term use of laxatives can set up a vicious cycle of bowel movements followed by constipation followed by further need for laxatives. The end result is that the muscular ability of the bowel to move waste along the tubes is weakened, causing more constipation and more pressure on the veins.

Avoid lifting heavy objects

If you cannot avoid it, try this. Bend at the knees without curving your back. Exhale as you lift up, breathe as naturally as you can while you hold the weight and then breathe out as you put it down. Definitely *don't* hold your breath when you lift the object.

Take more exercise

Walking, stretching and deep breathing all help to improve circulation and muscle tone, and reduce tension.

Tone those abs

A belly that sags towards the knees or hangs over the waistband is a sign of poor abdominal tone caused by weak muscles, and can predispose you to haemorrhoids. Regular keep fit, t'ai chi, pilates or yoga sessions are some of the best ways to tone and strengthen those abdominals. Or invest in a fitness video that includes special exercises for the abdominals. Or look out for women's magazines' fitness features for tips on how to trim that tum. And then introduce them into your daily routine. Simply reading about them and promising yourself you'll do it one day isn't enough!

Invest in a ring cushion

This is sometimes called a doughnut cushion, and it can make sitting more comfortable and creates less pressure on a haemorrhoid.

Don't scratch

Haemorrhoids don't always itch but if you're suffering:

- **Resist the temptation to rub or scratch.** This can cause a vicious cycle of itching and inflammation. Non-prescription haemorrhoid creams are designed to ease itching and pain. Anaesthetising creams and suppositories reduce inflammation. Ointments that contain hydrocortisone may help to decrease inflammation and speed healing, but they can thin the skin. Ask your doctor or a pharmacist. If you'd like to try more natural options, see herbal help (see next page).

- **Wipe gently.** Toilet paper can be irritating. You may find that soft tissues, 'wet wipes' that contain chamomile, cucumber or calendula, or make-up remover pads moistened with olive oil are soothing and more comfortable to use.

- **If itching persists?** There are many different causes for an itchy bum (medical term *pruritis ani*), so you may need to look for other possible causes such as fungal infection (common in the anal area), pinworm (see page 177), food irritants, tight or chafing clothing or laundry detergent/fabric softener residue.

Bathe regularly

Keep the anal area clean. Any excess mucus or faeces that remain after a bowel movement can cause irritation and inflammation, so washing after going to the toilet can be important for your comfort. Vigorous soaping of the anus can make itching worse because it disturbs the natural pH of the skin. A thorough sloshing and splashing the anal area with plain warm water, several times each day, should suffice and will help to reduce inflammation and irritation. Or you may find that using a shower, douche or bidet provides an easier way to clean up. Avoid flannel wash-cloths, ordinary soap, bath suds, shower gels and perfumes; these can all irritate.

> For more information on products, check out the Resource Directory on pages 323–328.

Get some herbal help

Herbal help for haemorrhoids and anal itching can include:

- **Aloe** (*Aloe vera*) is well known as a wound healer. When taken internally, this plant has a cleansing effect on the digestive system and is slightly laxative. Try Biogenic Aloe Vera Juice from Xynergy Health. As a topical treatment, aloe is cooling and healing. My all-time favourite is the pure and non-sticky Aloe 99, which I've seen work wonders on sunburn, scalds, leg ulcers and bedsores that refused to heal by other means.

- **Calendula cream** should soothe and reduce irritation. It's widely available under various shops' own-labels. My favourites are Nelsons, Neal's Yard, Jurlique, Kiwiherb and Spiezia Organic Calendula Ointment.

- **Witch hazel cream** or liquid (from chemists) acts as an astringent to reduce swelling.

- **Goldenseal** (*Hydrastis canadensis*) is astringent and healing to the gut wall. It soothes mucous membranes, helps the digestion and acts as a mild laxative.

- **Mullein** (*Verbascum thapsus*) calms inflammation and clears mucus.

- **Horse chestnut** (*Aesculus hippocastanum*) is a remedy often recommended for varicose veins and haemorrhoids. The active constituent, aescin, appears to strengthen blood vessels and reduce leakage. Try Aesculaforce drops or tablets from Bioforce or Horse Chestnut capsules from Viridian.

Give homoeopathy a go

It may be of value, especially if you've been suffering from haemorrhoids for a long time and the condition doesn't seem to be improving. Try homoeopathic Aesculus for burning haemorrhoids with a sensation of a lump in the anus that feels worse when walking, homoeopathic Aloe for haemorrhoids that throb, and homoeopathic Hamamelis for large haemorrhoids that are raw or bleeding.

Consider a course of acupuncture

It can be very effective at resolving congestion and stagnation.

Caution: if you're taking any anti-coagulant (blood thinning) drugs, such as heparin, check with your GP before using vitamin, mineral or herbal supplements.

Reducing the risk of piles

KATHRYN'S TOP TEN TIPS

1. Don't get constipated.

2. Don't put off visits to the toilet and don't strain when you get there.

3. Eat more dietary fibre.

4. Increase your intake of fresh vegetables and fruits, especially those with red and purple skins.

5. Drink more water.

6. Use suppositories and creams to relieve irritation and ease discomfort.

7. Learn to relax and let go. Follow the stress-busting advice on page 304.

8. See your doctor if you are suffering from any pain or bleeding.

9. Take daily exercise.

10. Remember that prevention is much less painful than cure.

WWW

Try the following websites for more information:
www.digestivediseases.org.uk/leaflets/piles.html
www.pilesadvice.co.uk

15.

What's Up?
Hiatus Hernia

Hiatus = opening; hernia describes 'an abnormal protrusion of an organ through tissue into another space'.

> **Read this chapter if you think you might have:**
> - Hiatus hernia
> - Acid reflux

Here we are with yet another health problem that is made worse by refined, rich food and lack of dietary fibre. Hiatal, or hiatus, hernia is where a portion of the stomach protrudes upwards through the diaphragm. What you may not know is that this common condition is a major cause of heartburn and can even feel like a heart attack. Left untreated, it can cause serious damage and may even increase the risk of oesophageal cancer. On the brighter side, there are people who have hiatus hernias but are never troubled by symptoms and only find out about them during unrelated X-rays or examinations.

Hiatus hernia types

There are three main types of hiatus hernia:

Sliding hiatus hernia

This is the most common type. A weakness of the muscles in the diaphragm can allow an upper part of the stomach wall and the lowest part of the oesophageal tube to stick up into the chest cavity. The upwards pressure pushes acid – and sometimes food as well – through the opening and back up past the oesophageal sphinctre, hence the feeling of heartburn or acid reflux.

'Rolling' or paraoesophageal hernia

A small percentage of hiatus hernias are known as 'rolling' (rather than sliding), or if you want to impress, learn to say paraoesophageal. Instead of sliding up into the oesophagus, this type of hernia 'rolls' upwards into the chest to lie alongside (that's the 'para' bit) the oesophagus. Because the area around the sphinctre isn't usually disturbed, acid reflux is less likely to occur with this kind of hernia. However, quite significant portions of the stomach can be pushed into the chest. If pockets of stomach sac fill up with gas, the pain and pressure can be really horrible.

It's easy to see why belching and vomiting are symptoms of this type of hernia. As the hernia gets larger, space normally available for the heart and the lungs is restricted. Sufferers can become severely out of breath and the heartbeat becomes irregular. The most likely treatment for rolling hiatus hernia is surgery to stitch the hole in the diaphragm.

Hernia in newborns

A much less common condition of diaphragmatic hernia is when, at birth, abdominal organs are found to protrude right up into the chest cavity. Usually diagnosed by X-ray, this is a life-threatening condition that requires urgent surgical treatment.

In more detail
Barrett's oesophagus is a relatively rare but potentially extremely serious condition that has acid reflux and regurgitation of food as two of its early symptoms. Read more about it on page 43.

The chicken or the egg

The link between hiatus hernia and heartburn is almost as undecided as the 'which came first' story. The medical opinion as to whether it's the hernia that causes the heartburn, or the sloppy sphinctre at the bottom of the gullet that causes the hiatus hernia, has see-sawed back and forth a number of times over the last few decades. As exploratory techniques have improved and endoscopes and gastroscopes have been able to get up close and personal with more and more of our important little places, the once-held view that almost every attack of heartburn was caused by a hernia shifted to the conjecture that, given the right circumstances, stomach juices could reflux into the oesophagus without there ever being a hernia present.

More recently, the new credo has become the old credo, so it is now believed that most cases of heartburn are, after all, caused by hiatus hernia. Back and forth and round and round we go. Well, they're not called medical circles for nothing! It now seems likely that, although slackness of that all-important sphinctre muscle is a factor, the trigger for most of the pain and discomfort we know as GORD or heartburn or dyspepsia or acid reflux might actually be – get this – a *small* hernia. In this case, small doesn't necessarily mean less serious as small hernias can still spew litres of acid and, yet, are more difficult to detect. So not only might they be missed; they might also be misdiagnosed. Accepting that there are also a number of other causes of hiatus hernia and of reflux, such as bad diet, poor posture, obesity or constipation, the jury is still out – so watch this space . . .

What causes hiatus hernia?

Causes or triggers of hiatus hernia can include:

Ageing
Constipation
Diets low in nourishment
Excess alcohol
Lack of dietary fibre
Being overweight
Poor digestion
Poor muscle tone
Poor posture
Pregnancy
Sedentary occupations
Shallow breathing

Smoking
Tight clothing
Unwise diet – spices, caffeine

Spinal misalignment – the very fact that, as humans, we stand on two legs instead of four, can put strain on the diaphragm and increase pressure.

Impact to or compression of the chest (resulting from an accident, for example) may also cause internal damage and trigger symptoms of acid reflux or hernia.

This is a long list and not all of it will apply to every sufferer. In very much the same vein as haemorrhoids, likely food triggers for hiatus hernia include the three Rs – Rich, Refined, Rubbish meals – low in bulk. These increase the likelihood of constipation and straining, put enormous pressure on the abdominal muscles and literally force the stomach upwards into the diaphragm. Such highly processed, nutrition-deficient diets, loaded with fats, sugars and dairy foods, also stimulate excess production of gastric acids, a scenario made still worse by obesity and the fashion for tight clothing.

Most likely symptoms?

Acid regurgitation at night
Difficulty swallowing
Gastrointestinal bleeding
Heartburn/acid reflux
Pain in the back, chest, shoulders or upper abdomen
Ulceration of the oesophagus

Action plan for hiatus hernia

The majority of hiatus hernia cases does not require surgery. But it can be important to undergo tests to rule out the possibility of other serious conditions. So if you've been suffering from the symptoms described in this chapter and have not consulted your doctor, then please do so. As well as consultation and examination, then he or she is likely to prescribe some kind of acid-suppressing medication. More on this on page 44.

The main aim of the dietary and lifestyle changes recommended here is two-fold: to reduce the symptoms of acid reflux and, at the same time, encourage your upwardly mobile stomach to stay where nature put it, below the diaphragm.

Better your digestion

Do whatever it takes to improve the way your body assimilates its food. What you eat is important but how you eat it and how you digest it is even more vital. Apart from improving your general nutrition, paying attention to meal mechanics can enhance transit time of food through the body. For the same reason, always stop eating before you're stuffed. Slow stomach emptying makes it more likely that the oesophageal sphinctre will relax, allowing gastric acids to go against gravity. If You Do Nothing Else . . . , starting on page 250, is the place for more information. In fact, it's essential reading for hiatus hernia sufferers.

Deal with constipation

A gunked-up colon puts pressure on the abdomen and the stomach, increasing the likelihood of reflux.

Eat more dietary fibre

You're probably fed up with my saying this but it really is one of the standard treatments for improving hiatus hernia.

Loosen that clothing

Slacken your belt and give up the girdle. If necessary, go up a size in clothing.

Snippets

A colleague has related an interesting case history concerning an elderly lady patient who presented with all the classic symptoms of hiatus hernia. As her treatment included acupuncture as well as nutritional advice, it was necessary for her to undress as far as her underwear. Layer after layer was removed until she stood there in the tightest bodice, complete with elastic sides and lace-up front. Asked if she really needed such a restrictive garment, the patient agreed that it might be superfluous to requirements and discarded it there and then. At a follow-up consultation, she said that all her symptoms had gone and not returned. It could have been the dietary advice and it might have been the acupuncture that did the trick, but it may also have been the casting aside of the corset.

Drink more water between meals

Yes, it's repetitive advice but I make no apologies for it. However, it's important to point out that too much fluid *with* food can make hiatus hernia symptoms worse by overloading and liquefying the stomach contents, which are then more likely to regurgitate.

Watch out for acid-forming foods

Cut back on items that are known to increase acidity, such as coffee, tea, meat, white flour and white sugar products, packaged meals and alcohol.

Deal with acid reflux

Follow the recommendations in the chapter on acid reflux (see page 36).

Take some exercise

There's no getting away from the fact that regular physical activity can help to improve the symptoms of this uncomfortable condition. But, for the reasons already explained, you need to choose your activity carefully. T'ai chi or regular keep-fit classes are good places to start. If you choose yoga, there are some postures that might not be suitable. If going out is a problem, why not consider investing in some home-exercise equipment? It doesn't have to cost a lot of money or take up heaps of room. For example, I have a stepper and a free-standing unit that looks like a cross between a treadmill and a 'ski' machine. Because they're both used in the standing position, there's no risk of aggravating a hiatus hernia.

I use each piece of kit for around five to ten minutes each day, so I know I'm always going to get at least fifteen minutes of good exercise, probably more, in addition to any walking or yoga that I might do. The whole lot takes up floor space of only about 1.5 × 1 metre (4 × 3 feet) and packs away flat when not in use. Walking and dancing (not jogging as it jars the spine and can aggravate acid reflux) are also excellent 'upright' exercises. If you cycle, either on a mobile or on a stationary bike, remember to sit up, not crouch over the handlebars.

Check your posture

This is so important. If you're not sure how yours is (good, bad or could be better), ask someone else to tell you. Crouching is for tigers not for humans with hiatus hernia. Try to avoid slouching, bending forwards or adopting any position where the stomach and diaphragm are restricted.

While your hernia is healing, forget about throwing a stick for the dog, playing racquet sports, lifting heavy weights or bundles, pushing heavy machinery or leaning down to clean out the bottom drawer, weed the path or wash the floor. If you need to be at ground level, sit down to the task and don't stay there for long. If you're a keep-fit enthusiast, this is one situation where toe-touching is off-limits.

Strengthen those abs

Exercises targeted at the abdominal muscles are essential to the healing of this condition. They improve the strength and tone of the diaphragm, so reducing the likelihood of acid backflow. A flabby abby, on the other hand, means poor muscle tone and the strong likelihood of equally poor bowel elimination and diaphragm function. Avoid repetitive sit-ups, which can put serious strain on the back and aggravate acid reflux. There's good fitness advice on strengthening exercises to be found in *Pilates – Creating The Body You Want* by Anna Selby and Alan Herdman. In the meantime, begin using the following breathing exercise.

Breathe

Shallow breathing is no help at all to a hiatus hernia. On the other hand, deep, slow, steady breathing can help to encourage the 'pinched' part of the gut to relax and go back where it came from. Don't be tempted to breathe in and out only into the chest. It can help if, when you breathe in, you deliberately push out your lower abdomen, not your chest. When you breathe out, try to 'roll' the breath so that your chest area 'bears down' towards your abdomen. There is a really helpful cassette tape called *Healthy Breathing* by Ken Cohen which has some easy-to-follow exercises. They're not specifically designed for hiatus hernia sufferers but are, nevertheless, potentially healing and strengthening.

Elevate the head of your bed

Raise it by 10 to 15 centimetres (4 to 6 inches). Make sure that whatever you use to raise it is solid and stable and not likely to slip. Or buy a purpose-made wedge that fits under the pillow end of your mattress.

Lighten the load a little

If you're overweight, shedding some of the excess could help ease your symptoms considerably. I've seen many patients lose all their symptoms of hiatus hernia and acid reflux when they lost weight. The advice under food combining (see page 283) may be of particular help to anyone reading this who has had difficulty shedding those extra kilos.

Try a natural antacid

For the occasional treatment of acidity, there are several drug-free remedies available. Silicea from Bioforce is soothing and protective, reduces inflammation and encourages healing of the digestive tract. Or try Gastroplex from Biocare (0121 433 3727) or Potters Acidosis tablets (from health food stores) for acidity that occurs after meals. Slippery Elm tablets, capsules or powder can reduce the risk of night reflux if taken with a little water an hour before bedtime.

Quit smoking

I've already said my piece on this subject and now it's up to you. If you need more help, I would highly recommend a fabulous little book by Dr Tom Smith called *Positive Options for Hiatus Hernia*. Apart from an excellent chapter full of extremely encouraging facts for quitters, there's also some seriously good information for all hiatus hernia sufferers.

Look after your liver and gall bladder

Naturopath, herbalist and author Dr Jonn Matsen (*Secrets of Great Health* and *Eating Alive*) believes that *unclean bile* can irritate the digestion, causing the stomach to spasm and put pressure on the diaphragm. Acid then leaks into the oesophagus, causing heartburn. His point is that supporting liver function might be a useful step if heartburn and hiatus hernia are present.

It's worth noting the importance of bile to the health of the digestive tract. It helps to stabilise the pH of the gut and acts like a natural disenfectant, encouraging good bacteria. Help your liver by going easy on the alcohol, giving your digestion a regular rest, avoiding artificial food additives, eating organic and only using medication that is really necessary. By the way, Dr Matsen is another writer who believes that humour is essential to health care. His books are excellent and I highly recommend them.

Get checked for Helicobacter pylori

Acid reflux can sometimes be associated with this ulcer-causing bacteria. Page 235 has more about ulcers.

> **Milk thistle**
> Milk thistle (*Silybum marianum*) is well known for its rejuvenating benefits to the liver. It has antioxidant properties and helps increase the production of new liver cells. Available in capsules but also as Milk Thistle tea with ginger and dandelion root from Biocare.

Deal with stress

Anyone with acid reflux or hiatus hernia knows that their symptoms can be a lot worse when they let themselves get wound up. That's because worry has a negative effect on the gut, tensing the abdominals, slowing down the digestion, constipating the bowel and causing us to lose control of the sphinctre that's supposed to stop the blow back of acid into the gullet. I've included a section later in the book that deals with stress and digestion which could be helpful to you. If you're interested, it's on page 304.

Consider the chiropractor

Or osteopath. Or physiotherapist. Spinal misalignment is believed by some practitioners to be a definite trigger for hiatus hernia.

For more information on acid reflux see page 36.

Reducing the risk of hiatus hernia

KATHRYN'S TOP TEN TIPS

1. Breathe more deeply.

2. Check your posture.

3. Cut back on coffee and alcohol.

4. Deal with constipation.

5. Drink more water between meals.

6. Exercise.

7. Improve your digestion.

8. Increase your fibre intake.

9. Loosen that clothing.

10. Lose a little weight.

16.

What's Up?
Intestinal Parasites

 Every patient with a disorder of immune function, including multiple allergies (especially food allergy) and patients with unexplained fatigue or with bowel problems, should be evaluated for the presence of parasites.
Leo Galland, MD, 1997

> **Read this chapter even if you *don't* think you might be suffering from intestinal parasites, and read it, too, if you think you have:**
>
> - Candidiasis
> - Chronic fatigue
> - Irritable bowel syndrome (IBS)
> - Leaky gut syndrome

OK, now here's a subject that most people would choose *not* to talk about, would prefer *not* to think about and don't, *for a second*, want to consider that they might be suffering from. The thought isn't made any easier when I remind you that one of the common names for parasites is worms. I expect you'll either take the view that this chapter is 'beyond the bucket' and you'd really rather not pursue it, or that it's interesting but couldn't possibly apply to you. So let's cut to the chase, stop beating about the bush and tell it like it is!

We all live with parasites!

A parasite is an organism that lives off the host – that's you and me – feeding either from our cells or from the food we eat. Like yeasts and bacteria, parasites can exist normally in the gut as long as digestion and elimination are working efficiently and there are enough digestive enzymes and friendly flora to keep them under control. But if the intestinal lining is damaged, production of acids, enzymes or bile salts is impaired or there aren't enough good gut bugs, then parasites can take hold.

How do you know?

If troublesome bowel symptoms are accompanied by persistent tiredness, an itchy nose or anal irritation – or if you have chronic fatigue syndrome (ME) or candidiasis, suspect parasites and deal with them accordingly. Do this anyway if diarrhoea-dominated irritable bowel syndrome (IBS) has not responded to any other form of treatment. Parasites are easy to miss and misdiagnose. For example, chronic giardiasis caused by the parasite *Giardia lamblia* can produce symptoms that mimic ME, leaky gut syndrome or candidiasis. Roundworm has been mistaken for a peptic ulcer. And because some parasites love to live off the sugar we eat, they can produce symptoms similar to those of diabetes or hypoglycaemia.

Don't freak out or feel embarrassed. Parasitic infestation is extremely widespread and a side-effect of being a human being. Parasites can live in our gut without any symptoms and may never bother us at all. But if they get out of hand, they can be the direct cause or trigger for a number of disorders that you may never have associated with parasites until you read this chapter. If you don't have them, the treatment will do you no harm.

Signs and symptoms

Likely signs and symptoms include:

Allergies	Itchy nose
Abdominal pain	Itchy skin
Bloated abdomen	Jaw clenching
Brittle fingernails	Joint pain

Broken sleep
Constipation
Cramps
Depression
Diarrhoea
Digestive discomfort
Disturbed appetite
Disturbed sleep
Fatigue
Flatus/gas
Food sensitivity
Foul-smelling stools
Frequent infections
Headaches
Irritable bowel syndrome
Itchy anus

Lethargy
Listlessness
Loose stools and episodes of
    constipation
Lower back pain
Low grade fever
Nails that show distinctly ridged
    longitudinal lines
Ravenous appetite
Skin irritation
Sugar cravings
Teeth grinding, especially at night
Unresolved candida symptoms
Weight loss

Or there may be no symptoms at all.

Beware
There are many causes of rectal or anal irritation that have nothing to do with parasites, including bubble baths and shower gels, talcum powder, over-zealous washing and the colours or bleaches used in toilet tissue and sanitary protection. An advice leaflet I picked up in a pharmacy suggests using 'a very soapy hand to cleanse the anus', and yet soap can be a common reason for itching. A couple of drops of tea tree oil swished into warm water and used as a douche can be just as effective and at the same time gentle. Or try using cotton make-up remover pads soaked with unperfumed cold-pressed oil (avocado, safflower or almond) to wipe the anal area clean. Sponges and flannel cloths harbour bacteria – don't use them unless they're hot-washed after every use.

If it's of any comfort, the chances of most human beings *not* cohabiting with some kind of parasite is trillions to one. Yes, I know we all know someone! But seriously, parasites are part and parcel of our life cycle. The human body supports a whole host of different life forms both on the outside skin and in the nooks, crannies and crevices of that extended doughnut hole, our inside skin. Most of these microscopic creatures do no harm. Some are actually beneficial; for example, the friendly gut flora that inhabit our intestines – part of our immune system's natural defence force – are absolutely essential for our health and well-being. There's a war going on down there all the time and the whole 'good guy, bad guy' battle is about keeping the balance in favour of those attentive, beneficial bugs. But sometimes, that stability is disturbed. When it is, our health is put at risk.

Old remedies, new attitudes

At least until the middle of the twentieth century, doctors would prescribe worm medicine routinely to anyone who was tired all the time. Parasites are still with us but modern medicine tends to ignore them and the misery they can create – probably because they are sometimes difficult to detect. The parasite's reproductive cycle, although prolific, can also be erratic, so that tests may come back marked negative even if parasites are still present. Available testing procedures can recognise only around fifty of the many hundreds of parasites that take up residence in humans. This means that tests catch about one in every five cases, which means that they're missing approximately 80 per cent of cases.

As to how many people are affected, statistics vary. A general consensus seems to suggest that at least 25 per cent of the population is affected. It's estimated that, at the current rate of spread, half the people of the Earth will pick up one or more parasites by the year 2025.

Unfortunately, parasitology (the study of human host parasites) is considered a problem of hotter climates, so training tends to remain the province of tropical disease departments in universities and teaching hospitals. This reasoning prevails despite the fact that parasites are no longer exclusive to areas of the world with tropical temperatures, poor hygiene or malnutrition.

So where do parasites come from?

Major reasons for the explosive spread of parasites in recent times include international travel, migration, easier importation of exotic foods, and the use and overuse of antibiotics. Parasites get into the body via several different routes and, if they like what they find when they get there (if our friendly bacteria levels are down or our immune system is compromised), they'll set up camp and make plans to multiply. If new settlements aren't kept in check, they spread and can become a serious and significant burden on the body. Major sources are believed to include raw fish, meat that isn't properly cooked, and produce that isn't thoroughly washed. Lack of hand washing, and contact with other people who are already infected, play a large part in the cycle of reinfection.

There are five main ways to pick up parasites or, more accurately, for them to pick on you:

1. Via food or water.

2. From an insect carrier such as mosquito, flea or housefly.

3. Through sexual contact

4. Via the nose, mouth and skin.

5. As a result of air travel to countries where parasites are endemic.

Once inside the body, parasites feed either on our food supply, in the digestive tract, or attach themselves and feed on us by sucking nutrients directly from our cells. These univited guests are pretty choosy. They select the best food and grow healthy, fat and randy while we survive on the leftovers. And they hang around, too. If left untreated, parasites can cohabit with their human host for years. It's perfectly possible that some-one might have eaten contaminated meat ten years ago and still be supporting a tapeworm population.

Types of parasite

There are lots of different types of parasites. In this chapter I've looked at five that commonly affect people living in the United Kingdom. Pin-worm, roundworm, tapeworm and hookworm all come under the family heading of Helminths. *Giardia lamblia* is a single-cell organism known as a Protozoa.

Pinworm

Known as threadworm in the UK, roundworm in the US, pinworm (*Enterobius vermicularis*, also known as *Oxyuris vermicularis*) is by far the most common worm infestation in temperate regions of the world. Depending on your source of information, it's been estimated that 20 per cent of children are affected at any one time, 90 per cent of all children are affected at some time or 100 per cent are affected most of the time. The most reliable data I can find seems to suggest that around 15 per cent of the total population (adults and children) is infected. In other words, whichever way you take the figures, pinworm is a prolific parasite. The UK name threadworm derives from the fact that the mature female worm resembles a short length of white cotton thread. Although this species is called roundworm in the US, it is not the same as the round-worm *Ascaris lumbricoides* that I mention further on in this chapter.

Pinworms are spread either by swallowing or by inhaling the eggs. Almost invisible to the naked eye, the eggs are laid at night as the adult worm emerges from the anus, tickling the skin as she moves around. The itching can be so severe as to disturb sleep. The sufferer scratches and the eggs either fall into the bedclothes or end up under the fingernails, whereupon they either pass to other people via any food that becomes contaminated or else find their way back into the body as the affected person touches their own face or puts unwashed fingers in the mouth or up the nose. Eggs that get back into the body via these routes – or those that climb back in from the anus – will hatch and continue the life cycle. I know you'll be thrilled, if you aren't already, to learn that one female *Enterobius* can lay as many as 10,000 eggs. Not all of these will mature but a great many will survive to adulthood and lay their own 10,000 quota.

Pinworms don't only congregate in the intestines but can also some-times be found in the vulva, uterus and Fallopian tubes when the worm loses its way after returning into the body after its nocturnal egg laying. This may be one of the reasons why pinworm infestation is more com-mon in women than in men. Women are also more likely to be involved in childcare, nappy changing, potty training and caring for sick children and, through housework, come into contact with the bedlinen and cloth-ing of everyone else in the family.

The chances of infestation are enhanced when we come to make the bed. As we straighten the bottom sheet or shake the duvet, eggs get onto our hands and fly into the air. Either they settle back into the bed, or we breathe them in, or they land on the floor to be picked up on bare feet, toys or anything else we put down there. You won't see them because they're so small, unless you happen to notice the hatched worms, those little bits of white string, around the back passage or in the stool. Other symptoms include itchy nose, itchy anus, ravenous appetite, broken sleep, bloated abdomen and general listlessness.

Pinworms are not life-threatening; but they are an unpleasant irritation that saps energy and becomes a drain on general health and well-being, not least because they compete with us for our food supply and deplete vital nourishment. In severe cases, they irritate the gut, causing pain that is similar to appendicitis. But by far the most harm is probably caused to our fastidious sensibilities. The immediate reaction to finding pinworm either in ourselves or in our children is disgust and an assumption that we're dirty. Living in too sterile an environment, especially as children, can compromise our immunity just as severely as exposing ourselves unwisely to undesirable bugs. But there is a balance and, in the case of parasites, good hygiene certainly helps to break the cycle. Surprising news to many people is that improving the diet can be one of the most useful treatments. Creating an internal 'terrain' that is healthy for us but hostile to the invader makes it more likely that any parasites will be discouraged or killed off by our internal protection forces.

First stop: the pharmacist

Medical treatment for pinworm is quick, easy and effective. Unfortunately, so is repopulation. Even if the recommended prescription of powder or tablet and follow-up dose is heeded to the letter, it only works on the worms that are currently in residence at the time. The tendency of human kind to scratch its bottom, pick its nose and suck its fingers leaves us particularly susceptible to picking up new eggs, and reinfestation is almost inevitable unless measures are taken to reduce the risk. The good news is that, although we may never avoid pinworms completely, we do develop a certain resistance to symptoms. In schools, it has been noted that some children build a strong immunity, while others continue to harbour persistent and recurring infestation. As in the case of all infections and infestations, parasites are most likely to invade and wreak havoc where general vitality is low – and this applies both to children and to adults. Parasites may be a factor in some of the health problems discussed in this book, including *Candida albicans*, irritable bowel and leaky gut syndrome. Some practitioners express particular concern that parasitic infestation is a special hazard to cancer patients.

Giardia lamblia

Giardiasis (and another prolific Protozoa infection, cryptosporidiosis) is most common in – although not exclusive to – countries where water quality and sanitation are poor. Although the precautions detailed in this chapter may seem burdensome or obsessive, they can significantly reduce the likelihood of your acquiring food-borne, water-borne or other parasitic infection.

Giardia lamblia is a bowel parasite that causes an intestinal infection known as gardiasis. I include it here because symptoms can be confused with those of candidiasis, chronic fatigue syndrome and leaky gut syndrome. *Giardia lamblia* is also sometimes, although not always, found in people with candidiasis. Symptoms can include foul-smelling flatus, watery, odorous diarrhoea, cramps, abdominal pain, bloating and burping. Untreated, severe cases can lead to malnutrition.

Giardia lamblia can be detected by microscopic examination of stool samples. However, identification becomes all the more difficult as the time between taking the sample and doing the test increases. It's important, therefore, that the lab receives and examines your sample within twenty-four hours. Even then, this is a parasite that sometimes just refuses to show itself, making it inconvenient but worthwhile to test three or four separate samples over a period of three or four days. In persistent cases, where stool samples continue to be negative, it may be necessary to arrange for a sample of the duodenal contents to be removed using an endoscope.

Giardia usually responds to the drug tinidazol (Fasigyn) or to metronidazole (Flagyl) but both drugs need to be carefully considered if you already have thrush or full-blown candidiasis which, you suspect, was caused by antibiotics in the first place! If tests are positive, discuss your concerns with your practitioner.

Giardia infection can be rampant in institutionalised care centres and day centres, where the parasite hangs around on surfaces such as tables, chairs, door knobs, stair rails, and so on. A doctor once told me that he believed one of the most bacteria-ridden places on Earth was probably a supermarket trolley. His reasoning? Children stand up in them with dirty shoes and people grab hold of the handles having just sneezed or picked their noses. Then, he said, we transfer the food that we put in the trolley onto our kitchen worktops and into our refrigerators. Yum.

Roundworm

Ascaris lumbricoides has been associated with human kind probably for all the centuries that we have associated with pigs. I'm referring to the porcine variety. These particular roundworms are the largest that live in the human gut. They look like earthworms, and can grow to over 30 centimetres (12 inches) long. They can live for up to a year in their favourite hidey-hole, the small intestine, feeding on undigested food. I imagine it could be this point where you decide to leave and move on but please don't because this could be important.

The damage caused by ascarids can be much more serious than that of pinworm. The single female roundworm can be responsible for laying anything up to a quarter of a million eggs every day. From the small intestine, the larvae penetrate the mucous membrane and are carried through the bloodstream to other parts of the body. Once in the lungs, they moult – twice – and then burrow out through the windpipe, gullet or throat. They return by whichever route is easiest for them, back to the small intestine. Maturing into full-size worms within ten to twelve weeks, the randy little gits breed like mad, only to begin the process all over again.

Apart from the obvious danger of malnutrition, this nasty round-the-body-and-back-again behaviour can lead to such proliferation that the worms can get tangled up and cause life-threatening blockages in any part of the intestines, plus severe infection including pneumonia. The worms are also suspected of giving off toxins that can cause behavioural changes. And if that wasn't enough, the body's immune system, in trying to fight off the parasites, produces antibodies that increase the risk of allergies.

I'm sure you'd like to know about symptoms. If only a few worms are present, there may be no obvious symptoms. As numbers increase so do the signs, which include abdominal discomfort, nausea, vomiting, irritable behaviour, loss of appetite, disturbed sleep, pneumonia and obstruction of the bowel.

Lack of hygiene must seem like paradise for these unappealing parasites because they're spread by hand-to-mouth contact and from human faeces. They're most common in the sub-tropics and rife in areas of the world where excreta is used as manure, or where there is open sewerage. But that doesn't mean that countries with good sanitation are exempt. Due to the expansion of foreign travel and exposure to areas of suspect hygiene most of us are probably going to come into contact with the not-so-little *Ascaris lumbricoides* at some time or other. Nor does it doesn't take any imagination to work out that imported produce from areas where the parasite is common could carry worm eggs. Another common source of contamination occurs during food preparation, emphasising the need to wash fresh produce. But, oddly, we often don't bother if things *look* clean.

A major reason behind the law that says catering workers must wash their hands after visiting the toilet, and before touching, cutting or cooking food, is to discourage the spread not only of bacteria but of parasites, too. Apparently, twiddling the tips of the fingers under a trickling tap does nothing to deter the single-minded ascarid. Only thorough and complete washing of the hands, including the fingernails, with hot water and soap will do. All the more vital, I know you'll agree, when I share with you the estimate that 98 per cent of the population either have roundworm in their intestines now or have had in the past.

Hookworm

Ancylostoma duodenale and *Necator americanus* are the unpronounceable Latin names for the two kinds of parasitic hookworm. Right away let me tell you that hookworm is rare in temperate climates, being most common in the tropics and rife where there is a lack of mains sewerage and poor diet, and where the population doesn't wear shoes. You thought ordinary roundworms were charming. Get a load of these guys. The life cycle is similar to that of its ascarid relation, above, but in this case, they get into the bloodstream by burrowing their way through the soles of the feet. Their common name comes from their habit of 'hooking' themselves to the gut wall, where they live off blood and mucus. They bite you and cause bleeding and necrosis (tissue death) of the intestinal wall. In severe cases, hookworm suck so much iron from the blood that anaemia results.

Hookworm is implicated in a vast number of stillbirths in third world countries, being a more severe complication during pregnancy than eclampsia. Individual worms can live as long as ten years.

Worm medicine works just as well for hookworm as it does for other types of parasite but, unfortunately, can be of limited use where reinfestation is inevitable. Proper sanitation and hygiene, including the wearing of shoes, are the best way to eliminate the risk.

Tapeworm

When I started researching the life cycle of the tapeworm, I actually wondered whether I should share its delightful antics with you or simply settle for the fact that it's a very unattractive multi-personality that you don't need to be acquainted with, tell you how best to avoid it or eradicate it, and leave it at that. But just in case you were ever infected, you'd need to know what was going on, so here's the low-down.

Human tapeworm infestation can come from the pig tapeworm (*Taenia solium*), the beef tapeworm (*Taenia saginata*) or the fish tapeworm (*Dibothriocephalus latus*). This tagliatelle-like parasite is actually a long ribbon of flatworms, all joined together from a common head, extended in segments to reach as long as 4 metres (13 feet) in the case of the pig worm, and 10 metres (32 feet) in the case of the fish worm. A single worm can be made up of between 3,000 and 4,000 segments, able to produce over a million eggs per day.

Each tapeworm segment is a separate individual containing both male and female reproductive organs. It hooks itself to – and feeds from – the gut wall. It multiplies when segments break off in the faeces and are picked up by other animals (referred to as intermediate hosts). As the larvae develop they travel to the animal's muscle tissue, where they form cysts. If this meat is then eaten, undercooked, the worm is released into the intestine of the new host and the cycle begins again. The most common sources of tapeworm to humans are fish and undercooked beef and pork, known as 'measly pork'. Dog tapeworm is transmitted from dog faeces and also when a dog licks your face or hands. Because tapeworm infestation interferes with the absorption of vitamin B12, it can lead to anaemia and may also cause fluid retention.

Tapeworms can be eliminated successfully using drugs. However, treatment can only be considered successful if the entire tapeworm is expelled. If the head remains, the worm will grow back.

Parasites also secrete toxins

Another disgusting habit of all parasites is that they produce toxins. By this means, a chronic parasitic infestation can put massive strain on the immune system, increasing the risk of other health problems, and also overworking the body's routes of detoxification that have to try to get rid of the toxins.

Action plan for intestinal parasites

This action plan is applicable to all types of parasite discussed in this section.

The whole tenet of natural medicine for parasites is to create an internal 'terrain' that is favourable to the host (you) and hostile to the parasite. However, a dose of speedy and effective worm medicine may be essential to remove unpleasant and potentially dangerous symptoms, in order to 'start with a clean canvas'. It's worth pointing out that dietary changes take longer to work and, in the case of, say, a serious round-worm or tapeworm attack, the sooner the little devils die the better. In the particular case of pinworm, which recurs so easily, the regular use of worm medicines can be very good at keeping it under control. However, I've talked with several practitioners who've raised a number of nega-tives concerning regular over-the-counter worm medicine: that it's not always effective for all types of parasite, that there can be side-effects such as headache and nausea, and that it's possible to become resistant to the drug. There's strong evidence to suggest that certain types of herbal medicine, together with improved diet and changes to certain lifestyle habits, may be far more effective at eradicating and preventing parasites.

If you suspect parasites

- Dose the whole family, using a preparatory worm medicine. Family packs are available in all pharmacies. If you're unsure about dosage, talk to a pharmacist. Don't be embarrassed. They get questions like this all the time. Repeat the dose according to the pack instructions – usu-ally around ten to fourteen days after the first one.

- If you decide to use homoeopathic or herbal worm medicine (see page 191), still treat the whole family. My suggestion would be to use the pharmacy medication as an initial treatment (above) and then use the homoeopathic or herbal remedies on a regular basis.

Reducing the risk of reinfection

Around the home:

- Change bed sheets regularly.

- Change towels and wash-cloths daily.

- Keep the floors around and under beds as clean and dust free as poss-ible (this simple housekeeping task can make a huge difference to allergy sufferers too).

- Leave outdoor shoes at the door and wear soft-soled shoes or slippers indoors.

- Don't walk around barefoot and then climb into bed without washing your feet.

- Wear underpants in bed during the period of treatment

- Wash your hands:
  - Thoroughly each morning, paying particular attention to under the fingernails.
  - Before preparing or eating food, after touching or playing with pets, or where there is coughing or sneezing.
  - After returning home from outside, especially after doing the weekly shopping.
  - Diligent hand washing is also one of the best ways to reduce the risk of catching or passing on a cold or flu virus.

- Wash all food produce, including fruits, thoroughly before eating.

- Change dishcloths, drying-up cloths and hand towels every day and put them through a hot machine wash.

- Especially during treatment, encourage children to wash their hands and to use disposable tissues if they need to sneeze or wipe their noses.

- Have family pets regularly wormed.

- Don't allow pets to lick your – or a child's – face.

Your diet

Improve the quality of your diet

Cut down on sugar, fatty foods and junk made with white flour. Introduce more fruits and vegetables and wholegrain cereals. Don't eat raw fish (sushi) or undercooked meat.

Eat pumpkin seeds

Add pumpkin seeds to salads or eat them on their own as a snack.

Use herbs and spices

Include lots of culinary herbs and spices such as rosemary, sage, thyme, turmeric, garlic and ginger in your cooking.

189

Drink vegetable juices

Juice fresh vegetables to make delicious savoury drinks. Try carrot, tomato, celery and/or onion. Onion juice is a traditional remedy for expelling worms.

Incorporate oils into your diet

Include two to three teaspoons of best-quality cold-pressed oils in your diet every day. Flaxseed (nutritional linseed) oil, hemp seed oil and pumpkin seed oil are good choices. Apart from providing you with valuable nutrients known as omega 3 and omega 6 essential fatty acids, these oils can help to reduce the risk of constipation and are believed to nourish and heal the digestive tract, and discourage parasites. Buy organic oils if you possibly can and always keep them refrigerated as they are very susceptible to damage by light and warmth. If you need oil for cooking, use extra-virgin olive oil, but don't heat other cold-pressed oils because doing so can damage their structure. Keep them for cold foods such as salad dressings, vegetable juices, smoothies and dips, for adding to soups before serving or for drizzling onto vegetables or just from the spoon. I love Viridian Pumpkin Seed or Hemp Oil, Green People Omega 3 & 6, Health From The Sun Liquid Gold Flax Oil (Arkopharma), Udo's Choice Ultimate Oil Blend (Savant) or any of the excellent cold-pressed oils from Higher Nature. Sadly, few supermarkets stock oils of this quality so try your local independent health food store or check the Resource Directory (see page 323) for stockist information.

Eat raw garlic

If you can tolerate it and enjoy it, add raw crushed (uncooked) garlic to salads, jacket potatoes, soups and vegetables just before serving. When garlic is cooked, it loses its parasite-deterring properties.

Take lemon juice

Fresh lemon juice in hot water first thing every morning is recommended in all cases of parasite infestation; so too is an infusion of lemon peel sipped at intervals during the day. To prepare the infusion, take one organic unwaxed lemon. Strip the peel (use a vegetable peeler) and steep it in a cup of boiling water until the water has cooled. Adults should chew and swallow the pips from fresh lemons and fresh grapefruit. But please note that pips are not considered safe for children in case of choking.

Eat foods that discourage parasites

Foods worth adding to your diet because they also discourage parasites include the following:

Cabbage	Linseeds
Carrots	Onions
Cranberry juice	Papaya (paw paw)
Fennel	Pomegranate
Figs, fresh or dried	Pumpkin seeds
Fresh pineapple	Sage
Lemons and grapefruit	Thyme

Your personal health

- Treat constipation (see pages 80–95).

- Improve transit time by improving digestion (see page 250).

- Wash the genital area thoroughly after emptying the bowels and before and after sexual intercourse.

Eating outside the home

- Avoid sushi and salad bars, street food, and restaurants that don't wipe the tables or have flies buzzing around.

- Don't take bar nuts or nibbles. The fingers that dipped into them before yours may not have been washed.

- Remember that ice makers use unfiltered water. Freezing may kill parasites but not bacteria.

Some useful remedies

Homoeopathic medicines

For pinworm in children, try homoeopathic Cina 6C or Teucrium or Nat. Mur (two four times daily away from mealtimes).

Garlic cloves

A freshly peeled garlic clove, inserted anally at night and left until the next bowel movement, helps to kill worms that congregate in the rectum. I've heard and read several times that garlic cloves were fashioned in this shape specifically for this purpose but have no research to back it up! Lubricating the clove with pure aloe vera gel or garlic cream helps insertion. Repeat every night for two weeks. Garlic may not be enough on its own to despatch parasites but it can be a useful adjunct to other treatments and is almost certainly a deterrent to reinfestation.

Did you know?

All these plants have anti-parasitic properties and can be used in various combinations to help discourage parasites. However, never be tempted to self-medicate using raw plant material or to self-prescribe home-made herbal tinctures. It's worth pointing out that anything that is strong enough to kill a parasite could also be concentrated enough to harm the person taking the medicine. The wrong dosage or the wrong combinations could be as dangerous as taking the wrong drugs, so I would caution you to use only prepared proprietary medicines, follow the instructions and take only the stated dose. The plants highlighted in bold are provided with further descriptions below.

Barberry bark	Fennel	Pumpkin seed extract
Black/green walnut	Garlic	Sage
Chaparral	Goldenseal	Tansy
Cinnamon	Grape seed extract	Thyme
Cloves	Oregon grape	Turmeric
Cranberry extract	**Papaya**	**Wormwood**

Black walnut

This is sometimes called green walnut, and it is rich in the minerals chromium and iodine. Black walnut is multi-talented. Apart from being anti-fungal and anti-parasitic, it helps to oxygenate the blood (hugely beneficial given that parasites hate oxygen). It can eradicate parasites from blood and lymph fluids and also from organ sites such as the brain, heart, kidneys, liver and intestines. And it's blessed with laxative properties, which help to expel parasites once they have been killed off. Black walnut aids in expelling tapeworms and pinworms and may also be of use in the treatment of candidiasis symptoms.

Wormwood (Artemesia)

This is a traditional treatment for parasites and is used in some areas of the world to treat malaria. It helps to maintain the natural ecology of the intestinal tract, and can relieve gas and soothe the abdominal gripes associated with parasites. It's said that wormwood can sufficiently anaesthetise a worm for it to lose its grip on the gut wall and be more easily eliminated.

Cloves

Clove extract is another plant medicine with a long history in the treatment of parasites. Cloves are also strongly antiseptic and anti-bacterial. Unfortunately, a great many spices are irradiated, which destroys these properties. Cloves used in anti-parasitic medications should therefore be from non-irradiated sources.

Papaya

Papaya fruit extract is good for – or should I say bad for – parasites because it helps to digest them. Papayaforce tablets taken regularly after meals can eradicate parasites and also act as a digestive aid. I am advised by the makers, Bioforce, that Papayaforce is safe for children as well as adults.

When choosing remedies always choose top-quality products from recognised suppliers. I've heard good reports of Barberry Plus from Biocare and Paraclens from Higher Nature. Green Walnut tincture, Wormwood and Clove capsules are also available from G&G Vitamin Centre.

Use probiotics

Repopulate the gut flora with probiotics. Parasites thrive in the absence of proper intestinal flora. Creating a healthy terrain by replacing the good bacteria is just one of the ways of discouraging parasite reinfestation.

Practitioner help

Where parasites are suspected but seem resistant to treatment, or where symptoms are not improving, I would very strongly recommend a consultation with a nutrition or naturopathic practitioner who is familiar with the treatment of candidiasis, gut dysbiosis and parasites. Reduced levels of stomach acid, insufficient digestive enzymes or an imbalance of gut flora can all predispose to parasites. Stool samples, taken over three-day intervals, can be analysed and will confirm whether or not parasites are a problem.

Reducing the risk of parasites

KATHRYN'S TOP TEN TIPS

1. Dose regularly with worm medication.

2. Try homoeopathic or herbal remedies.

3. Keep hands away from bottoms and noses.

4. Wash hands thoroughly and frequently.

5. Change bedlinen, towels and wash-cloths often, especially during an attack.

6. Don't walk around with bare feet.

7. Invest in a regular course of probiotics.

8. Eat lots of fresh fruits and vegetables, but wash them all thoroughly before use.

9. Avoid raw fish and rare meat dishes. If they are served undercooked, don't eat them.

10. When dealing with worms, remember that the best treatment is prevention, creating conditions in the gut that discourage the parasites from setting up home there.

For further information on parasites **www.DrHuldaClark.org** and **www.anti-parasite.com** have interesting pages on parasites and their treatment.

For the more scientific aspects, go to the United States *Centers for Disease Control & Prevention* at **www.cdc.gov** and search 'parasites'.

17.

What's Up?
Irritable Bowel Syndrome

❝ Surveys have shown that over 40 per cent of patients who visit internists do so for gastrointestinal problems. Half of those have 'functional' complaints. Their gut is malfunctioning but no one knows why. No anatomical or chemical defects are obvious. . . Their gut is thus acting up in such a way as to defy the best that modern medicine has to offer, which in this case is ignorance compounded by lack of compassion. ❞

The Second Brain, Michael Gershon, MD, 1999

> **Read this chapter if you're suffering from irritable bowel syndrome (IBS), or if you have:**
>
> - Diarrhoea
> - Constipation
> - Gallstones

Don't ever be persuaded that irritable bowel syndrome, familiar to most of us as IBS, isn't a genuine or serious condition. Nothing could be further from the truth. The unfortunate thing about IBS is that it's terribly misunderstood. It is also very frequently misdiagnosed. You can have it and yet it might be completely overlooked. Or you may *not* have it but you're told you *do* have it. IBS has become the all-encompassing acronym for almost any collection of bowel symptoms that have no obvious cause, but for which all other gut disorders have been ruled out. Many's the time that real sufferers don't get the acknowledgement they deserve or the treatment they need, while a whole load of other people get labelled with a condition they actually never had in the first place. Don't be too keen to blame the doctor, though. There's no medical test yet available that can establish whether you have IBS, so all he or she has to go on is your list of symptoms plus the results of a range of test results that have excluded all other possible causes.

Until quite recently, it was believed that IBS was nothing more than a psychosomatic disorder. Reports of patients being referred for psychiatric or psychological assessment were not uncommon – and yet this condition is a long way from being 'all in the mind'.

An interesting piece of research

One report told the tale of a group of IBS patients who waited an average of seven years before a firm diagnosis of their condition was made. In an investigation carried out at the University of Edinburgh Gastrointestinal Unit, the case notes of six IBS sufferers were examined. Five of the six were referred for psychiatric assessment – although none was actually diagnosed with any psychiatric disorder. They each saw a minimum of six different specialists, yet many of the hospital doctors involved were not aware of the investigations already carried out elsewhere. Between them, these patients underwent a range of major operations, with one person being sent for surgery seven times, another six times.

What is IBS?

Irritable bowel syndrome is defined as a 'non life-threatening disorder of the gastrointestinal (GI) tract, involving muscular spasm and inflammation in the large colon, abdominal pain (recurrent and often severe), and a pattern of alternating diarrhoea and constipation, for which no organic cause can be found'. IBS is also classified as over-reaction or excessive nervous stimulation of the digestive system and the large intestine in response to emotional triggers. There may be pain on eating which is relieved by a bowel movement. Stools may be mucusy, loose and liquid, ribbon-shaped or pellet-like.

In a nutshell, if you have IBS, your digestive system could be fairly described as hyperactive, hypersensitive and dysfunctional. IBS won't kill you but, say some of the sufferers that I've spoken to, the symptoms can make you feel as if you want to die.

Internal explorations including barium meal X-ray and colonoscopy do not usually reveal anything to be seriously wrong. Most times, the intestines are found to be completely healthy apart from being in a state of constant motion (no pun intended) characterised by excessive rumbling and gurgling – known as borborygmi, and some tenderness when examined.

Confusingly for the person who has it, IBS has several other names, including colicky bowel, nervous bowel, mucous colitis, mucomembranous colic, non-inflammatory bowel disease, nervous diarrhoea, spastic constipation and spastic colon. I think it might be better described as a 'spasmic colon'.

What causes IBS?

It's difficult to talk in terms of what causes IBS because, unfortunately, no one can really be sure. But there are plenty of identifiable triggers and lots of life situations, emotional, physical and environmental, that can aggravate the condition. Such as:

Being physically run down or feeling emotionally low
Bowel infection
Candida albicans
Chemotherapy or radiotherapy treatment
Disorders of the nervous system
Drug side-effects
Food sensitivity or intolerance
Gynaecological problems
Inadequate digestive enzymes
Intestinal parasites
Low levels of stomach acid
Nutrient deficiencies
Poor digestion
Poor-quality diet
Relationship conflicts
Some types of iron supplement, such as ferrous sulphate
Stress
Surgery
Work pressure

A major characteristic is fluctuating transit time. When food travels too quickly through the system, it's pretty obvious that it isn't going to be fully digested. The undigested particles then irritate the gut, causing it to empty suddenly. Fierce episodes of diarrhoea can be followed by a period of intestinal impasse when, in response to the excessive bowel activity, everything literally solidifies – that is until the next episode of manic movements.

IBS can co-exist with premenstrual syndrome, plaguing the sufferer during the week before a period. And IBS has also been associated with a disorder called fibromyalgia – painful and inflamed tendons, muscles and ligaments and chronic fatigue – described as 'having a whole-body headache'. Symptoms may be worse during an IBS attack – and vice versa. Experts have yet to determine the reasons for any link but one suspect is deficiency of serotonin (see opposite), which is already abnormally low in people with fibromyalgia and is known to fall even lower during times of bad weather. IBS flare-ups sometimes coincide with changes in barometric pressure, as they also do in fibromyalgia. I wonder if it might also be significant that 90 per cent of this 'brain' chemical is manufactured in the bowel?

IBS is sometimes misdiagnosed as diverticulitis – and vice versa. The two conditions are quite different, but IBS may lead to the formation of diverticula (see page 105) if the diet is too low in fibre.

The symptoms

Intermittent or dominant IBS symptoms may include:

Abdominal pain	Exaggerated reflexes
Anal soreness or irritation	Flatus
Anxiety	Headaches
Backache	A feeling of incomplete evacuation
Bleeding	Incontinence or leakage
Bloating	Lethargy
Borborygmi	Mucusy stools
Constipation	Nausea
Cramping	Painful periods
Diarrhoea	Panic attacks
Erratic heartbeat	Proctalgia fugax – intense rectal pain

Rapid breathing   Weight fluctuations

Teeth clenching   Vomiting

Tiredness

> ### Jargon buster
>
> **Serotonin** is a neurotransmitter, responsible for transmitting information from one nerve cell to another. It is also known as a natural mood elevator and tranquilliser and is often found to be low where there is chronic pain, depression, migraine, food cravings or insomnia.

The role of stress in IBS

Although stress can be a significant factor in IBS, it doesn't mean that any of these symptoms are all in the imagination. It simply indicates that stressful experiences exert an unusually powerful physical effect on certain brain chemicals and hormones. Like crossed wires at the telephone exchange, mixed-up messages are sent to the intestines, where peristalsis (muscular contraction of the gut) is over-activated, triggering the bowel to empty more frequently.

Most exciting for the IBS sufferer is the more recent acceptance of a long-held theory that the bowel has its own thinking and messaging service known as the enteric nervous system (ENS). This gets talked about as the 'bowel brain' because it's believed to be the only part of the body that can control reflexes (such as bowel emptying) without any input from the 'head brain' or the spinal cord. This new research brings IBS into the realms of real diseases and affords it the respect that it deserves.

Family stresses and strains

Some IBS sufferers complain of being dominated by relationship conflicts (often with parents) where they may feel suffocated or trapped. Where constipation is dominant, there may be a reluctance to 'let go', to give anything away. Where diarrhoea has the upper hand, some people express fear and loneliness bound up with over-anxiety. And as appears to be the case in many bowel disorders, there may be stored anger and unexpressed feelings.

Recommended reading

If you're interested in the psychological aspects of physical illness these books may be of special interest:

Frontiers of Health by Dr Christine Page (C.W. Daniel). I'd class this as an exceptional read. Highly recommended.

Also worth delving into are *The Healing Power of Illness* by Thorwald Dethlefsen and Rudiger Dahlke (Element), and the now extremely famous *You Can Heal Your Life* by Louise L. Hay (Eden Grove).

Ask your doctor

It's important to obtain an accurate diagnosis. Food allergies, gluten intolerance, lactose intolerance, Crohn's disease, ulcerative colitis, endometriosis, colon cancer, ovarian cancer, diverticulitis and gallstones are just some of the conditions that share symptoms with those of irritable bowel syndrome and need to be ruled out before a definite IBS diagnosis can be made. If part of the digestive tract has been surgically removed (for example the stomach or part of the small intestine), the resulting increase in transit time or, in the case of gall bladder removal, the malabsorption of bile, can impersonate the desperate diarrhoea associated with IBS.

If you haven't been offered any tests and your symptoms don't seem to match those of IBS but you're still told that 'it's probably IBS' because the doctor can find nothing else wrong with you, then I'd say either ask for a second opinion or change your doctor.

VERY IMPORTANT POINT

If you suffer from IBS and have been advised by your doctor or a specialist to eat more bran, read about fibre first (see page 271).

Action plan for irritable bowel syndrome

Encouragingly, there are several gentle yet effective approaches to the management of an irritable bowel. The two most important corner-stones are:

1. To isolate the foods that are likely to cause you the most grief and either find suitable substitutes or introduce new ways of eating so as to make the agitators less troublesome.

2. To do whatever it takes to deal sensibly with stress. By disturbing the nervous system and the adrenals, anxiety and worry have a direct and negative effect on the intestines. Sometimes, stress can trigger an attack all by itself. At other times, it may be stress and food together. A food that is normally not a problem when life is calm and snag-free could become a trigger food if you happen to eat it when you're steering your way through a particularly stressful day.

Your diet

Increase your fibre intake

The rules about roughage apply a little differently to anyone with IBS. You can't just throw a load of bran at the breakfast table and expect IBS to go without a fuss. For a start, anyone with a touchy intestine of any kind should treat wheat bran and any other wheat-based foods – such as bread, cakes, biscuits, pastry and pasta – with extreme caution. Research that has been confirmed by considerable feedback from patients seems to suggest that wheat bran irritates more than it soothes. I think that the most useful advice I could give you right now is to concentrate on those foods that have higher ratios of soluble fibre (see my note about this in Chapter 22 on dietary fibre), and include insoluble fibre only in tiny amounts to test for sensitivity.

Avoid artificial sweeteners

They can cause severe gripe and may trigger attacks of diarrhoea. Avoid them by reading pack labels and saying no to anything that contains artificial sweeteners including sorbitol, candarel/aspartame and saccharin. Be aware that many packaged foods labelled with the word 'diet' contain sugar substitutes.

Beware

Foods to avoid if you have IBS

Artificial sweeteners	Excess alcohol
Carbonated drinks	Fried and fatty foods
Chemical food additives	Non-organic chicken and eggs
Coffee	Red meat
Cow's milk	Wheat bran
Custard, puddings and creamy desserts	

Steer clear of sugar

As I've mentioned elsewhere, sugar is a nutrient-robbing non-food that, in my view, will do you no health favours. However, it's worth repeating here that, when it comes to IBS, there's some disagreement as to whether or not sugar makes symptoms worse. Many leading naturopaths and nutrition experts agree that a diet high in refined sugar may be a highly significant contributing factor to IBS, primarily because a rapid rise in blood sugar levels can effectively 'paralyse' the rhythmic contractions of the small intestine, slowing down the progress of food and allowing gut bacteria more time to feed off the sugar. It's well known that, of all the dietary components, carbohydrates (and that includes sugar) have a major impact on intestinal bacteria and gas formation.

There are others, though, who believe that simple sugars cause no problem to most IBS sufferers. Heather Van Vorous, author of two specialist books on irritable bowel syndrome and herself a former sufferer, points out that 'sugar should not become a major component of your diet' and has 'zero nutritional value', but she is also adamant that 'one of the best things about the IBS diet is that it requires no restriction of sugar'.

I see this conflict as yet further confirmation that diet is a peculiarly personal thing and that what suits one person well will drive another's symptoms off the scale. I've met IBS sufferers who fit both profiles, some being upset by sugar and others apparently not bothered by it at all. My advice would therefore be to keep sugar to an absolute minimum, at least while you are going through the recovery process, and then to introduce sweet foods occasionally as treats. If you need to use sweetening, best-quality honey can be a better option than ordinary sugar.

Watch out for chemical E-numbers

Anything that smacks of artificial preservatives, colourings or flavours is a potential trigger for IBS. Become an avid label reader. Steer clear of unnecessary additives (most of them are completely unnecessary). Say no to products that include E-numbers, fillers, binders, emulsifiers, modified starches, lactose and fructose. Make your food from basic ingredients so you know what goes into it, and choose as many organic foods as you can.

Say no to fizz

Carbonated drinks are a definite no-no for IBS sufferers. Not only do the bubbles push loads of gas into the intestines, but they may also contain artificial additives (watch out for sweeteners here too) and copious quantities of caffeine. Carbonated water can be a useful digestive aid for some people, but it isn't good for IBS. Still mineral water, herbal teas and soups are not only healthier but kinder to the gut.

Drink plenty of water

Do this between meals (see page 289).

Stay off the coffee

It's well known for its laxative action. If you have a sensitive digestion, coffee can give you abdominal cramps and an urgent rush for the loo. And no, sorry, decaff is not the answer. Caffeine is just one of around 500 chemicals in coffee, some of which are suspected of causing cramping, the last thing you need if you've got IBS. Honestly, it's best avoided altogether. Get a taste for dandelion coffee, Bambu coffee substitute or herbal tea. Your gut will be grateful.

Go easy on the cow's milk

It seems to be a real hard-to-digest food for some IBS sufferers so I'd suggest taking it in very small amounts (organic milk only) or finding an alternative. Research shows that avoiding lactose (the natural sugar content of milk) can help to relieve symptoms. Lactose is often used as a food additive so it can also be worthwhile checking packet labels. There's more on lactose intolerance on page 215.

Removing milk from your diet does not mean that your bones are likely to fall apart. There is heaps of research worldwide that shows there's little or no benefit to calcium levels from cow's milk. In fact, your body uses up calcium and magnesium as it tries to reduce the over-acidic conditions caused by the milk protein. Not only are there absolutely loads of other really excellent sources of calcium in a wide variety of foods (see page 217), but there are also a great many delicious dairy alternatives, including soya, rice and oat milk. Spend an hour or two researching in your local health food store. You'll be amazed.

Avoid fatty and fried foods

They don't help IBS either. Butter, margarine, spreads, suet and shortening should all be avoided. Anything that makes the digestion work harder is likely to worsen IBS symptoms. Fats are slow to digest. Low-fat foods are very often loaded with chemical additives. Although extra-virgin olive oil, and nut and seed oils, are healthier options, it's an unfortunate fact that oils can trigger an attack just as easily as solid saturates. So by all means include the healthy oils but use only small quantities.

Give up red meat

One of the worst IBS trigger foods, red meat is a tough one to digest. You may think that because you don't notice any particular symptoms the burger, the chop or the steak has done nothing but provide you with a good protein meal. But beef, pork, lamb and game take an extremely long time to be broken down, and in the process put huge strain on all parts of the digestion. As they chug their way, oh so slowly, through the intestines, meat products putrefy (go off) and expel toxins that irritate the gut. And how they irritate! If you're not convinced that avoiding the meat is a good move, then give it up just to avoid the antibiotics and hormones, and other less than desirable ingredients that still find their way into intensively farmed meat and poultry feed. Drug residues are serious suspects in the hunt for IBS triggers.

What about booze?

Whatever your state of health, overdoing the alcohol is a dull move. Alcohol is strong enough to irritate not only the digestion but all body systems, and it isn't just IBS sufferers who can be upset by it. It's just that they may notice the symptoms more immediately. You'll probably already be aware whether or not alcoholic beverages send your gut into overdrive. If they do, then they're best avoided. The main rule for drink is don't do it on an empty stomach. And definitely don't drink spirits, beer, lager, liqueur or sherry. The exception is vodka, being the purest alcohol; splashed with a little soda water, it's an option if your IBS is candida-related. An occasional glass of dry wine (red or white) seems to suit some sufferers. Once again, the only way to find out is to experiment.

Go organic on eggs

IBS sufferers may find that the fat in egg yolk is enough to trigger an attack but egg whites usually pose no problems. In my view, there is nothing to merit the use of mass-produced eggs. So if you use eggs, go organic free-range.

Get the best from fruit

Anyone familiar with my books or articles will know that I usually recommend that we eat a lot more fruit and that we should consume it on an empty stomach. This works extremely well for most digestive disorders, and in particular for dyspepsia, hiatus hernia and acid reflux. It's even helpful for some cases of IBS. But for others, it simply doesn't work. So here are some tips to help you make the best of your fruit:

- Always discard the skin. The fibre in it is just too hard to take and, unless its organic, will be a rich source of pesticide residues.

- Chop, slice or juice your fruits. Either combine them with a protein drink, or have them after an oat or rice cereal breakfast, or after a main meal, rather than before it.

- Fruit salad is usually best digested if taken as a starter but if you have IBS, try it as a dessert instead.

- My feedback from former patients is that rhubarb, plums and oranges can be severe IBS triggers and may be best avoided altogether.

- Fruit juice poured into an empty as well as sensitive system can trigger urgent bowel emptying. Packaged orange juice may be the worst culprit. I'd say don't buy it.

- Other juices, such as those made from apple and grape, can also aggravate a sensitive system if they are taken when the stomach is empty. This is one of those situations where juice is best mixed with soya milk or blended with a banana, or taken after meals rather than before food.

- Cranberry juice is a good accompaniment to your daily spoonful of linseeds (see page 278). Avoid cranberry that has added sugar. Biona Organic Cranberry is sugar-free and should be available from health food stores.

Experiment with nuts

Unless of course you are allergic to nuts, they are a seriously nutritious food, full of healthy monounsaturated and polyunsaturated oils, dietary fibre and vitamins and minerals. However, the insoluble fibre in nuts, together with their high fat levels, can make them a difficult food for IBS sufferers. The only way to find out if they agree with you is to experiment with small quantities. One way to make them easier to digest is to grind them and mix them into drinks and desserts or sprinkle them over salads or into yoghurt. If you grind them to a paste, they make an excellent spread for rice cakes or rye crackers, and if blended with water they can be turned into a useful 'milk'.

Eat vegetables right

Vegetables are nature's superfoods, packed with protective antioxidant nutrients and that all-important dietary fibre. For IBS sufferers, though, the insoluble fibre content of vegetables can be a serious trigger. In addition, the Brussels sprouts, cabbage, cauliflower, calabrese/broccoli family breaks down into sulphur compounds that give off copious quantities of gas. The humble onion and all its relatives – leeks, garlic, shallots – do the same. Rather than avoiding vegetables altogether, try a few tips that may make digesting them much easier:

- Cook vegetables a little longer than you are normally advised to. Al dente may be healthy, but not if it sends your digestion into explosive spasms for days on end.

- Chew vegetables really well.

- If you love salad, eat it at the end of a meal instead of as an entrée.

- Make lots of vegetable soups. Liquidising or blending cooked vegetables breaks down the fibrous bits so they are easier for your digestion to deal with. The bonus is that you get lots of extra nutritious fluid and achieve your daily quota of vegetables at one meal.

- Mashing your greens, especially Brussels sprouts and broccoli, improves their digestibility.

- Well-cooked baby spinach leaves may be easier to digest than raw salad spinach.

- Avoid corn (maize) in all its forms. It's great for fibre content, but for IBS sufferers it's positively gut-ripping.

Improve the digestibility of beans

Beans (legumes) are notoriously gas producing. But as is the case with some vegetables, mashing them or adding them to blended soups can improve their digestibility. If you cook your own beans from scratch, make absolutely certain they are fully and properly cooked, and that you skim the pan and change the water several times during the soaking and cooking process. The foam produced during cooking isn't called 'flatulence foam' for nothing. If you use canned beans, buy organic, then rinse them thoroughly through a sieve before use to discard the liquid they're packed in.

Practise better digestion
Do whatever you possibly can to improve the way your body deals with the food you give to it. Page 250, *If You Do Nothing Else* . . . has a list of essentials.

What about good foods for IBS?

The only way to really find out which foods agree or disagree with you is to experiment. This list isn't exclusive but has been compiled from my own patient feedback.

Almond milk

Basmati rice

Carrots

Chickpeas

Egg white

French sticks

Hummus

Low-fat yoghurt (sheep's or
   goat's milk)

Noodles

Nut butters

Oat milk

Oatmeal and oat bran

Organic chicken

Pasta

Pitta bread

Potatoes

Prawns

Quorn products

Rice Dream

Sourdough bread

Soya cheese

Soya protein

Soya milk

Sweet potatoes

Textured vegetable protein (TVP)

Tofu

Tuna in spring water

Vegetable soups

White fish

One of the best ways to increase the range of foods in your diet is to spend an hour or two browsing in your local independent health food store and seeking out dairy-free and wheat-free alternatives. You'll be surprised at the variety available.

Pills, powders and prescriptions

Among the most likely prescriptions for IBS are:

- Anti-cholinergic/anti-spasmodic drugs, designed to block the messages that trigger increased motility of the intestines and reduce spasms.

- Direct-acting smooth-muscle relaxants that have directly calming effects on the muscles of the gastrointestinal tract.

- Peppermint, which is both antispasmodic and what herbalists call carminative (calming). It is much used in the treatment of IBS. However, be aware that some peppermint-based drugs and peppermint supplements can aggravate acid reflux conditions.

- Laxatives to relieve constipation (see page 88).

- Bulking agents. These may contain ispaghula/psyllium, methylcellulose, bran or sterculia. They are often referred to as laxatives, but a more accurate description would be 'fibre supplements'. Their aim is to increase the volume of the stools by absorbing water, so softening the faeces, making them just as helpful at treating and preventing diarrhoea as they are in relieving constipation. Psyllium can be used every day without risk of overdose or dependence. A pharmacist or your doctor should be able to recommend isphaghula/psyllium-based products. If you have supply problems in the UK, the food supplements companies Solgar and Higher Nature have some excellent psyllium-fibre products in their catalogue. Colon Care (Blackmores or Biocare) or Ispaghula capsules (Arkopharma) are useful if you are away from home.

Did you know?

Psyllium and ispaghula (*Plantago ovata and Plantago ispaghula*) have been used as safe and effective laxatives for thousands of years. Closely related plants native to southern Europe, the Mediterranean, Pakistan and India, they grow well wherever there are dry, open spaces.

Psyllium seeds and husks have high levels of soluble fibre, which expands and takes on a gelatine-like appearance when in contact with water. This bulks the stools, reducing their density and easing the passage of waste through the large colon. The gentle behaviour of psyllium stimulates normal peristaltic activity without causing cramping or griping. Psyllium also helps to break down the build-up of mucus and undigested proteins in the gut, making it a valuable natural, drug-free, internal cleanser that encourages the removal of putrefactive toxins from the intestines. Psyllium's adaptogenic and regulatory action also makes it a useful supplement for the treatment of diarrhoea and haemorrhoids. *Always take any fibre supplement with lots of water.*

Psyllium also contains essential fatty acids and is often recommended as a dietary aid for reducing cholesterol. If you spot the word 'isphagula' on food packaging, that's because it's sometimes used as a stabiliser.

Beware

A great many prescription drugs contain not only artificial colours but also artificial sweeteners. Do check labels and ask about side-effects, as chemical additives can seriously aggravate some cases of IBS.

Supplements that may help

Multi-vitamin/mineral complex

Take this daily in your new healthy eating programme. Brands that are high on my list of favourites include Viridian, Biocare, Solgar and Blackmores.

White Willow Complex

Available from Biocare, this contains a range of herbs that are known for their ability to settle and soothe the digestive tract. Golden seal has anti-inflammatory properties. Echinacea is famous for increasing resistance to infection, but may also help digestion and reduce flatulence. The liquorice content soothes mucous membranes. Grapefruit seed extract has anti-bacterial and anti-fungal properties. And the white willow itself contains salicin, another herbal anti-inflammatory that seems to calm an unsettled stomach and intestines.

Gastroplex

This is also available from Biocare, and can be a useful supplement to help ease some of your symptoms while you're waiting for a diagnosis. Take it with White Willow Complex (above).

Globe artichoke (Cynara scolymus)

Shown in studies to ease the discomfort of IBS, reducing abdominal pain, cramps, bloating, flatulence and constipation, cynara supplements are widely available. Try Cynara capsules from Lichtwer Pharma or Arkopharma.

A nourishing and soothing snack

Add a small carton of sheep's or goat's milk yoghurt to half a cup of organic soya milk, a whole banana and two teaspoons of linseeds or psyllium powder to make a delicious smoothie that can help to ease both constipation and diarrhoea.

Probiotics

A regular course of probiotics should be considered essential for IBS sufferers. A number of studies has shown them to be helpful in relieving diarrhoea, aiding the digestion of lactose and improving general gut functioning. There are some excellent brands of 'good flora medicine' available. My top choices include Blackmores Acidophilus & Bifidus, Biocare Bio-Acidophilus, Viridian Tri-Blend Probiotic Powder and Solgar's Advanced range of Probiotics. Quality probiotics are also available from Ecozone and Higher Nature. I'd suggest a three-month course at least once a year and *always* as a follow-up after antibiotics. Page 294 has important information on the health benefits of healthy gut flora and the Resource Directory (see page 323) has stockists.

For more information on supplements, check out the Resource Directory on pages 323–328.

What else can you do?

Ask for help

Consult a practitioner who is familiar with natural treatments for IBS. If at all possible, arrange to have tests to help rule out candida and parasites (see page 70).

Avoid smoking

The chemicals in cigarettes are known to over-stress the digestion and can have an urgent laxative effect on the bowels – not something to encourage, especially if you suffer with IBS-related diarrhoea. If you live or work with smokers, try to get them on your side and explain that passive smoke could be worsening your condition.

Get rid of stress

If you're exposed to excessive stress you need to take extra-special care of yourself. Living with stress is not good for your physical or emotional health. Your IBS symptoms may be a sign that your system signalling for help. Do something about the problem before it overwhelms you and you develop something more serious than an irritable bowel. If you've suffered severe emotional trauma that could be affecting your health, you could benefit from seeing a clinical psychologist. Talk to your doctor about a referral. And don't be afraid to ask: the service is there to help you. Rest assured that you're not alone and you're not the only one who feels this way – you're certainly not 'going mad' or 'losing it'. Everyone is affected by fear and trepidation; it's simply that some of us are more susceptible than others.

If your IBS is stress-triggered, the Jan de Vries Bowel Essence might be worth a try. I'm also a great fan of Arkopharma's Californian Poppy capsules, which soothe the rough edges on those days when nothing is going right. They're non-addictive and don't cause drowsiness, but do help to relieve tension – and they are a good remedy to take if you have difficulty relaxing. Try them with Arkopharma Ispaghula fibre capsules. Blackmores Celloid Magnesium Compound can ease stress and anxiety and is excellent for bowel cramps.

Take some exercise and relaxation

If exercise and relaxation are going to be beneficial, they need to be enjoyable. They definitely *don't* need to be either complicated or time-consuming. Choosing the right programme can do so much to help you unwind and to encourage a calm colon. Fifteen or twenty minutes a day is all it takes. If you can spare an hour a day, then so much the better. Yoga and t'ai chi both combine exercise with relaxation. Try a local class that emphasises relaxation and deep breathing (check out the tape mentioned on page 314), or if this isn't convenient, go for a beginners video tape that you can follow at home. Taking leisurely walks every day in the fresh air is healthy, relaxing and free. Unless it's gale force and torrential, don't be put off by a bit of inclement weather. Just wrap up warm under a waterproof coat and go for it. Don't see a wet day as a foul day. Rain is just nature's balance for fine weather. The world is just as beautiful behind the clouds.

Get plenty of sleep

It's worth pointing out that sleep deprivation is used as a method of torture. It's not a pleasant thought, but it reminds us all how important sleep is for our health and well-being. Get a few early nights. Take a book or some music with you and lose yourself. Five-minute catnaps during the day can be calming and regenerating, too. If sleep eludes you, try a herbal remedy. I would choose Nitebalm drops, available from Natural Woman, Arkopharma's Valerian Capsules or Passiflora Complex from Bioforce.

Try complementary therapies

Although there is very little in the way of medical or scientific research to support their use, there is strong and positive patient feedback on the benefits of aromatherapy, reflexology, Indian head massage and shiatsu in helping to reduce tension and stress.

- **Meditation** is a highly recommended method of gaining your own space and quietening your mind. It takes practice but do persevere; the results are worth the time and effort. Your doctor should be able to refer you to a qualified practitioner.

- **Traditional Chinese Medicine (TCM)** using acupuncture and herbs has also been shown to be especially helpful for IBS. In TCM, anger and worry cause stagnation of energy in the liver and spleen, resulting in gastrointestinal dysfunction. Some patients have reported that their condition improves following sessions of spiritual healing.

- **Hypnotherapy** has an excellent track record in the treatment of IBS. A study carried out at the University Hospital of South Manchester, England (and reported in the *Lancet* in July 1992) found that hypnosis had a calming effect on the gut, reduced pulse rate and slowed the breathing.

Recommended reading

IBS Diet by Sarah Brewer with Michelle Berriedale-Johnson (Thorsons).
Irritable Bowel Syndrome & Diverticulosis by Shirley Trickett (Thorsons).
Food and the Gut Reaction by Elaine Gottschall (Kirkton Press) has an
  excellent recipe section.
The Sinclair Diet System by Carol Sinclair (Vermilion) also has good
  recipes. A helpful approach if starchy foods make your gut problems
  worse.

Reducing the risk of IBS

KATHRYN'S TOP TEN TIPS

1. Choose soluble fibre first; treat insoluble fibre with care and respect.

2. Make mealtimes special and take your time.

3. Eat fruits, salads and vegetables at the ends of meals.

4. Chop, mash or liquidise fruits and vegetables.

5. Always discard the peel from fruits and vegetables.

6. Steer clear of high-fat foods.

7. Drink plenty of uncarbonated water between meals.

8. Do more exercise, including Kegels (see page 92).

9. Set aside some quiet time for yourself each day.

10. Get lots of rest.

www.eatingforibs.com is the website of Heather Van Vorous, a food writer who specialises in creating recipes for people with IBS. Her book *Eating For IBS* is practical and sensible. As a fellow sufferer, her advice comes from the heart. 'If your doctor doesn't take your symptoms seriously', she tells us, 'get yourself another doctor. It's up to you to educate [them], and then dump them if they persist in their ignorance at the expense of your health. You deserve support, concern and consideration for what is a very genuine and serious problem.'

Hear! Hear!

Eating For IBS by Heather Van Vorous is published by Marlowe & Company.

Also worth visiting are:
www.ibsnetwork.org.uk
The IBS Network, St. John's House, Hither Green Hospital, Hither Green Lane, London SE13 6RU.

18.

What's Up?
Lactose Intolerance

> **Read this chapter if you have problems digesting milk.**

If you suffer from lactose intolerance, you're definitely not unusual or alone. Some estimates suggest that more than three-quarters of the world's population (including many people of oriental, Asian, Arab, African, Jewish and Latin/Mediterranean descent) is unable efficiently to digest cow's milk. Indeed, pasteurised milk products are simply not part of the natural staple diet in most areas of the globe. So widespread is the condition that one might say that 'lactose tolerance' is the unusual case and 'lactose intolerance' a normal state of affairs.

What is it?

Lactose intolerance, also sometimes called hypolactasia, disaccharidase deficiency or dairy product intolerance, occurs when there is a deficiency of an enzyme called lactase, which is needed to break down lactose, the natural sugar content of milk. The condition may be inherited (known as primary intolerance) or acquired due to a digestive disorder, stomach surgery, infections or ageing. As we grow older, our bodies tend to produce less and less lactase.

What are the symptoms?

Likely symptoms include:

Abdominal bloating	Nausea
A feeling of fullness	Diarrhoea
Abdominal cramps	Smelly stools
A build-up of intestinal gas	Mucusy stools

When lactose is allowed to pass through the digestive system untouched by lactase, it's left to the friendly *Lactobacillus* bacteria to do the digesting. (The same kind of bacteria are used outside the body to make yoghurt from milk.) Unfortunately, it's often the case that those with digestive troubles are already low in friendly bugs. The upshot is that any leftover lactose is likely to be leapt upon by not-so-friendly gas-forming little devils who belch and fart around inside your gut, leaving abdominal bloating, colic and diarrhoea in their wake!

Notice how similar those symptoms sound to irritable bowel syndrome (IBS). I have seen quite a few patients who were convinced that they had IBS improve 100 per cent simply by cutting down on cow's milk. Interestingly, many were still able to eat some types of good-quality cheese and yoghurt (see page 218).

Some people can handle small amounts of dairy foods but others may find that their only option is to avoid them completely. Where the production of lactase is limited but not lacking completely, the condition is sometimes referred to as lactose maldigestion. The difference between this and lactose intolerance is that maldigesters with reduced supplies of lactase can still digest some milk products. In addition, if there is an ample supply of friendly *Lactobacilli* bacteria in the gut, some milk sugar will be broken down even if the lactase enzyme isn't there. But as disturbed gut flora is common in those with digestive difficulties, this doesn't always happen.

Milk and calcium

The argument that because milk is rich in calcium it must be a good calcium source for humans seems irrefutable. Milk is, indeed, a rich source of calcium – which is great news for calves whose stomachs are designed especially for it, but not so great for people who are unable to digest it.

Several reports show that, lactose apart, cow's milk intolerance can cause serious damage to the mucous membrane lining of the human gut. Milk has also been implicated in asthma, runny nose and glue ear, excess production of stomach acid, IBS, diarrhoea and arthritis. Long-term studies suggest that those who do go back to consuming milk in adulthood may later develop other problems, including asthma and eczema.

It's also a common misconception that cow's milk is the *only* worthwhile calcium source for humans. This is definitely not true. There are lots of non-dairy foods that provide valuable amounts of this important mineral, including:

Blackstrap molasses
Brown rice
Canned sardines, pilchards and salmon
Carob flour
Dried fruits
Fortified soya milk
Nuts, especially almonds, Brazil nuts and cashew nuts
Oats
Pulses
Sea vegetables such as hizike, wakame and nori
Sesame seeds and tahini
Sunflower seeds
Tofu

The majority of vegetables and herbs contain some calcium. Good sources include:

Broccoli, especially the stalks	Onions
Brussels sprouts	Parsley
Cabbage	Parsnips
Carrots	Swede
Dandelion leaves	Taro leaves
Drumstick leaves	Turnips
Fenugreek	Turnip tops
Kale	Vine leaves
Okra	Watercress

Many people who are intolerant of milk are sometimes still able to take (properly fermented) yoghurt, buttermilk, fermented milk drinks such as Yakult™ or Bio-Danone™ and some real cheeses, especially those that are made from sheep's or goat's milk, rather than cow's milk. This is because some or all of their lactose content is broken down during the fermentation process, making them easier to digest and, as a bonus, making the calcium content more 'bio-available' to the body. It's worth noting that yoghurt consumption is often high in countries where the population doesn't drink pasteurised milk!

Beware

Whatever your degree or level of lactose intolerance, avoid these cheeses and all types of ice cream:

Cottage cheese	Ricotta
Feta	Processed cheese
Gruyere	Cream cheese
Mozzarella (pizza cheese)	Ice cream
Neufchatel	

As well as the items listed above, avoid all kinds of cow's milk, whether dried, UHT, fat-free, skimmed, semi-skimmed or full fat.

Watch out for hidden lactose in:

Prescription and over-the-counter medicines. Tell your doctor and the pharmacist if you have a problem with lactose.

Spreads, dips and dressings

Desserts and sweet treats

Packaged and canned soups

Cereals

Biscuits, buns, breads and cakes

Any foods that mention casein, caseinate or sodium caseinate, curds, lactoalbumen, lactoglobulin or whey

Supplements that *don't* tell you the product is free of lactose, whey and sugars

If you have low levels of lactase rather than a complete deficiency and enjoy cheese, it's worth knowing that some cheeses have more lactose 'pre-digested' during the curing process. However, try them in small amounts to test for tolerance:

Brie	Gorgonzola
Camembert	Gouda
Organic Cheddar	Monterey
Cheshire	Port Salut
Dry curd cheese	Roquefort
Edam	Stilton
Gloucester	Wensleydale

Dairy-free labels worth looking out for include:

Vitasoy	Rice Dream
Provamel	Rakusen's
Plamil	Trufree
Oatly	The Stamp Collection

Delamere Direct has a range of goat's milk products, and St. Helen's Farm supply goat's milk products to some major supermarkets.

Pretreated milk

If you're lactose-intolerant but really love milk and don't want to give it up, you can purchase lactase supplements that allow you to pre treat your milk so that the lactose is digested before consumption. Or you could take a capsule with meals that contains the milk-digesting enzyme. Lactose-reduced and lactose-hydrolysed milks are also available. If you're eating out and are worried that there may be hidden lactose in any foods, take a lactase enzyme capsule with you.

Note that while the above products are certainly useful for some people, I have found that they are not always helpful to those with chronic intestinal disorders such as candidiasis, IBS or leaky gut syndrome (LGS), or where there is poor liver function.

A regular course of probiotics (see page 294) can also help to reduce the symptoms of milk intolerance.

My own research, reading and experience in practice has convinced me that cow's milk is usually tolerated in small amounts but is best avoided by most of us. If your digestion is dodgy or your bowels bothersome, either avoid cow's milk altogether or keep it to a minimum and make sure that what you do buy is organic. Look for the lowdown in If You Do Nothing Else . . . on page 250, which also includes some good alternative sources of calcium for those who cannot manage cow's milk and are worried about calcium intake.

See your doctor

If you identify with the symptoms I've described in this chapter, give up dairy products entirely for three days. If the symptoms disappear and then come back again when those foods are reintroduced, then I would strongly suggest that you see your doctor for a check-up. There are several tests available for lactose intolerance, including blood, breath and stool tests.

More good reasons to give up milk

I have copied the following, with kind permission, from the excellent newsletter *Food Matters At The Inside Story*. The original was taken from the *Vega Review*. VEGA (Vegetarian Economy and Green Agriculture) is a charitable organisation that monitors current intensive farming and food production. For more information or to take out a subscription, contact VEGA, 14 Woodland Rise, Greenford, Middlesex UB6 ORD. Telephone: 020 8902 0073; website: www.vegaresearch.org

> Despite the fact that margins have fallen to the point that dairy farmers can scarcely cover their costs, the average dairy cow is being worked ... harder. Her average annual output has risen from 4,950 litres in 1984 to over 6,000 litres today. She is now culled after four lactations (at age 5) whereas a cow of this type kept without commercial exploitation could expect to live for up to 20 years. During her short life she has a . . . 35% chance of suffering from mastitis – (painful) inflammation of the udder caused by bacterial infection, stress and physical damage. Her udders become hot and hard with abnormal discharge . . . normally accompanied by lameness in one or both hind legs and swollen joints. . . . To achieve this high milk yield, she will be artificially inseminated every year. Her milk is too valuable to be wasted on her calf from whom she will be separated when it is a few days old – separation from her calf is potentially the most distressing incident in the life of a dairy cow.

Forcing production in this way, especially if hygiene is not a top priority, may cause her udders to become painful and so heavy that they drag on the ground resulting in frequent infections and over-use of antibiotics.

Recommended reading

Food allergies (see page 115).

Check out the following for further information:
www.stamp-collection.co.uk has information on dairy-free products and links to other good sites.
www.dialspace.dial.pipex.com/town/park/gfm11/ contains more information on lactose intolerance.

19.

What's Up?
Leaky Gut Syndrome

❝ The preservation and restoration of normal intestinal permeability rests on two principles: building resistance and reducing risk. ❞

The Four Pillars of Healing, Leo Galland, MD, 1997

Read this chapter if you suspect that you have:

- Candidiasis
- Food allergies
- Gluten sensitivity
- Intestinal parasites
- Irritable bowel syndrome (IBS)

Got a gut like a sieve? Well you could have and not even know it. If the gut wall gets damaged, we may suffer from a condition known as leaky gut syndrome (LGS), sometimes called intestinal permeability. This strange-sounding problem is very common. If you're unlucky enough to be affected, it can be the cause of allergic reactions and a long list of other nasty symptoms. If you already have another bowel or digestive disorder, intestinal permeability could be making it worse, or might even have caused it in the first place.

Although not readily acknowledged by conventional doctors, leaky gut syndrome is considered by many naturopaths and nutrition-oriented doctors as a major cause of disease. It has been implicated as a contributing factor in cases of the following:

Arthritis

Asthma

Candidiasis

Chronic fatigue syndrome (ME)

Chronic sinusitis

Crohn's disease

Depression

Eczema

Fibromyalgia

Food allergy/sensitivity

Headaches

Irritable bowel syndrome

Lupus

Migraine

Premenstrual syndrome

Ulcerative colitis

Jargon buster

Leaky gut syndrome is defined as: 'An increase in permeability of the lining of the intestines to large food molecules, antigens (foreign invaders) and toxins, leading to inflammation, cell destruction and mucosal damage.' In plainer language, the gut gets full of holes that allow undigested food, bacteria and toxins to leak into the bloodstream.

It's like this

You'll remember from our journey through the digestive system (see page 10) that once foods arrive in the small intestine, they're broken down ready for absorption through the gut wall into the bloodstream. The barrier between the gut and the blood is already full of holes, even in a healthy person, but the openings are of a particular size, designed to allow certain desirable molecules to pass through and to keep out the undesirables. They act a bit like a sieve or strainer with very tiny perforations or, if you prefer, a series of locked gates to which only certain substances have the right keys. In an undamaged gut, many vital nutrients are absorbed via this route.

So, if the holes get bigger, doesn't this mean that you can absorb more nourishment? Unfortunately, no. When the membrane becomes inflamed, ulcerated or otherwise damaged or eroded, large molecules of food leak through to the lymph system and general circulation before they have been properly digested. The immune system doesn't recognise these large bits of food and thinks they're aliens – because, of course, under healthy conditions, they should be a lot smaller. So the alarm is raised and the body sets about trying to chase them away – hence the allergic reactions associated with the condition. In the process, oxygen and fuel are used up, ultimately driving the system itself to exhaustion. Not surprisingly, sufferers of leaky gut syndrome become severely fatigued and more susceptible to infections than they would otherwise be.

It's also important to remember that most nutrients don't just sit there alongside the gut wall and then soak slowly through into the blood. In the case of minerals, for example, they have to wait to be attached to a protein which then carries them across. But when the lining is damaged, the protein carriers get damaged too and can't do their job. So, as well as everything else, you, the host, become prone to vitamin and mineral deficiencies.

If that weren't enough already, the inflammation caused by leaky gut syndrome also harms the antibodies that help to protect us against viruses, bacteria and other invaders. Immune cells wear out and can't be replaced in sufficient numbers. In fact, cells throughout the system don't get the nutrients they need to work efficiently. They also become toxic because the normal detox pathways are damaged and wastes don't get carted away. The havoc that this creates isn't hard to imagine. Just think what your daily life would be like without proper fuel or waste disposal.

Picture having a whole lot of buildings made of Lego but not being able to dismantle them into the pieces that you need to make other structures. This is what happens when food isn't properly broken down into the building blocks that are needed for repair and renewal. The nutrients from a supper of, say, salmon and salad which might have been used by the body to repair that cut on your finger, replace some worn-out cells in your liver, or help protect you against that cold virus you breathed in yesterday, don't get absorbed in a usable form. It's perhaps an oversimplified analogy but you get the picture.

The inflammation that results from the creation of all this garbage in turn produces free radicals, rogue molecules that can reduce our immunity to disease. Free radicals are well capable of making even more holes in that already damaged intestinal wall, perpetuating the leakiness of 'leaky gut syndrome'.

It's also likely that if you have this condition you'll find yourself increasingly intolerant of a greater number of foods. I guess it's a bit like vandals squeezing through the gap in a broken fence, poking tongues at the gardener and trampling on the vegetable patch – ultimately destroying the food supply. What can also happen is that the poor old battered gatekeepers trying to protect the 'fence' against further injury by producing a mucus barrier along the gut wall only make things worse by overcompensating, blocking the pathway with excess mucus and further hindering the absorption of nourishment.

What causes LGS

Because of the vicious circle that connects leaky gut syndrome with candidiasis and food allergies, it's hard to know which of these conditions comes first. It could be the overgrowth of invasive yeast getting through the intestinal barrier that causes the 'leaks'. Or perhaps something else, such as an allergen, damages the lining and this then allows *Candida albicans* – the yeasty beastie that we look at on page 65 – to do its worst. It's certainly the case that bits of undigested food floating around and decaying in the gut can create the perfect conditions for bacteria, *Candida* and parasites.

As more foods arrive, hoping in vain to be properly digested but instead just providing food for the bad guys, the gut wall is continually irritated and becomes even more permeable. More yeasts and toxins flood through, and so the cycle begins again. If the cycle isn't broken, all that happens is that the next meal – and the next – produces more bloating or discomfort or sensitivity.

Likely causes or triggers

Any one of the following could aggravate or even kick-start leaky gut syndrome:

Gluten sensitivity (see box, page 226)

Inadequate levels of stomach acid

Insufficient natural antihistamines (possibly due to poor absorption or deficiencies of certain nutrients)

Intestinal parasites

Lactose intolerance

Misguided use of medicines, especially antibiotics, steroids and non-steroidal anti-inflammatory drugs (NSAIDs)

Poor food combinations

A consistently poor-quality diet, high in fats, sugars and refined foods

Ongoing and unrelenting stress

Reduced liver or adrenal function

Rushed eating habits

Stomach upset, gastroenteritis or viral infection

Compromised immunity

Exposure to high levels of pollution

Heightened sensitivity to pollution

Inadequate digestive enzymes

Some specialists are convinced that faulty digestion of carbohydrates (starchy foods and sugars) is responsible for the initial injury to the absorptive surfaces of the intestine, increasing the likelihood of a damaged and leaky gut. This could explain why changing to a low-carbohydrate diet can often help to reduce the symptoms of bowel and digestive disorders, especially during the healing process.

In more detail . . .

Gluten is a sticky protein found in wheat, rye, barley and oats. In the condition known as coeliac disease, the gluten causes permanent injury to the cells in the intestinal walls and, for this reason, people suffering from the condition have to follow a gluten-free diet.

It is, however, possible to be sensitive to this gluey protein even if you do not have coeliac disease. Although there are as yet no definite answers as to why gluten is able to cause such damage, researchers have turned their attention to the interaction of the starch and protein components of gluten-containing grains. Flour granules have a starchy centre surrounded by a protein coating – the gluten. It may be the interaction between the starch and the protein that leads to the incomplete digestion and absorption and causes intestinal gas, diarrhoea, bloating and abdominal discomfort.

Research also points to the possibility that a carbohydrate molecule in the gluten might contain toxic properties capable of causing direct damage to the gut wall. Unabsorbed carbohydrates comprise one of the most likely sources of gas in the intestines and are a potential source of distress not just to sufferers of coeliac disease, but also to those who have parasitic infestation, irritable bowel syndrome, candidiasis, and food sensitivity, as well as leaky gut syndrome. Several of the symptoms of coeliac disease are similar to those of other gut disorders. The actual flattened and blunted appearance of a damaged gut membrane is also common to a number of different conditions.

It's interesting that some nutrition experts have long seen gluten as a major culprit in slowing down the passage of food through the gut and have considered it to be responsible for much bowel discomfort in non-coeliac sufferers, too. Significant improvements have been noted where gluten-rich foods have been kept to a minimum or avoided altogether.

The symptoms

Likely symptoms of leaky gut syndrome include:

All the symptoms of candidiasis (see page 65)
All the symptoms of intestinal parasites (see page 177)
Bloating
Chronic fatigue
Irritable bowel syndrome
More susceptibility to viruses and bacterial infections
Poor digestion
Sensitivity to a range of foods
Weakened immunity

The emotional and psychological side

The inability to digest and absorb nourishment has been linked by psychologists to a reluctance to digest or absorb new information or changes. It also seems that some people with digestive or absorptive problems may feel 'sour' about something, allowing conflicts to 'eat them up inside' rather than expressing their feelings. They may also suffer from mind wandering and poor concentration. This could apply just as easily to, say, ulcers or acidity as to leaky gut syndrome.

What can you do?

Allergen-free diets are a first-line treatment in helping to heal a holey intestine. Continual exposure to allergens can simply sabotage any worthwhile treatment. It's also vital to treat candidiasis and parasites, and to take all possible steps to improve the digestion.

In addition, there are several specialist non-drug products that have shown good results. These are recommended for use under practitioner guidance. As in the case of candidiasis (see page 65) and parasites (see page 177), if you think that leaky gut syndrome applies to you, I would very, very strongly suggest that you seek a consultation with a therapist who is familiar with LGS and candidiasis and their nutritional treatment. It's a complicated condition that shouldn't, in my view, be tackled without professional support. Most experts agree that symptoms need to be dealt with in a certain order if they are to be eradicated. Leading nutritionist Gillian Hamer of London's Wren Clinic recommends that, if candida is present, it should be controlled before attempting to heal the gut wall.

Find a nutrition-oriented practice

You may need to travel but the effort should be worth it. Ask in your local health centre. Health food shops are often a good source of information. Go by recommendation. When you find someone, ask to talk to other people who have been treated by the same practitioner. Don't be afraid to ask about their qualifications. Ask about the tests that are available to check for candida and parasites. If the practitioner concerned doesn't know about them or can't provide them, I'd strongly suggest finding someone else. There's more information in the Resource Section (see page 323).

Action plan for leaky gut syndrome

While you are waiting for an appointment, this action plan may help to reduce symptoms.

Your diet

Avoid common food allergens

Especially cow's milk, eggs, wheat cereals, bread, corn and nuts.

Avoid gluten

By removing wheat products and bread, you will be eating much less gluten, the sticky allergic protein that I talked about on page 226, but there is also some gluten in oats and rye.

Avoid refined foods and yeast

Cut out all sugar artificial sweeteners, coffee, foods made with white flour and anything containing yeast (bread, beer, stock cubes, cake, bought dressings).

Avoid all alcohol

At least while you're trying to sort out your symptoms.

Reduce your intake of hormone and antibiotic residues

By avoiding non-organic meat and poultry. Organic lamb is well tolerated by most meat-eaters. Choosing the organic option whenever you can also helps to reduce your intake of pesticide residues.

Reduce the risk of parasites

Never eat raw fish or underdone meat, and follow the advice given in Chapter 16.

Eat sheep's or goat's milk yoghurt

If dairy products are not a problem for you, eat a small carton of sheep's and goat's milk yoghurt every day. Buy small quantities with an advanced 'use-by' date. Use them up quickly and then buy new supplies. The fresher the product, the more friendly bacteria it is likely to contain. Always keep yoghurts refrigerated and transport them from the store in a chill-carrier. Don't use cow's milk products of any kind if you have leaky gut syndrome.

Become an avid label reader

Make every effort to avoid packaged foods that contain artificial colourings, flavourings, preservatives, emulsifiers and stabilisers. If a packet contains all these things, ask yourself :

a) is it real food?

b) do I need it?

What else can you do?

Steer clear of cigarette smoke

(Again!)

Replace the good bacteria

The chapter on friendly flora (see page 294) explains why and how.

> **VERY IMPORTANT POINTS**
>
> **Treat for candidiasis**. Not everyone with leaky gut syndrome will have been overrun with *Candida albicans* but the chances are high (see page 65).
>
> **Treat for intestinal parasites** (see page 177). Most people with LGS/candidiasis are affected by parasites.
>
> **Check out the chapter on food allergies** (see page 115). Some of the information there may be relevant to you.

Take plenty of exercise

Physical activity encourages detoxification; it's vital in a toxic condition like leaky gut syndrome. Rebounding (mini-trampolining) is especially highly recommended – it's a way of 'jogging' without jarring the spine. Dancing, aerobics, keep fit, yoga, t'ai chi, chi gong, cycling, rowing, golf or just plain old enjoyable and cost-free walking are also good. Exercise to sensible limits. Don't exhaust yourself. And don't work out on a full stomach.

Build up a sweat

It's a powerful way to cleanse the body, especially of accumulated pesticide residues and industrial toxins.

Drink right

Replace the fluid you lose through sweating. And drink plenty of filtered water every day, especially between meals.

Avoid unnecessary medicines

Do this unless the medicines are essential for your survival. *Don't* stop any prescribed drugs without consulting your medical practitioner but do find out if your prescription is really necessary. Heart drugs, thyroid or diabetic medication would be considered essential, for example, but you may be able to manage without antacids or painkillers. NSAIDs, for instance, have been linked to leaky gut syndrome. Talk to your doctor.

Take some remedies

To help diminish the impact of food that may not be properly broken down, fifteen minutes before each meal take half a teaspoon of Enteroguard powder (Biocare). Enteroguard contains fructooligosaccharides, which encourage the growth of friendly bacteria; vitamin C, which is believed to stabilise mast cells and reduce the release of histamine that is produced in response to the allergic reaction; and N-Acetyl Glucosamine to help repair the damaged gut lining. Some candida experts also recommend Butyric Acid Complex, also from Biocare (one capsule three times daily with food), because it acts as a support to friendly bacteria and helps to heal the gut wall.

> **Jargon buster**
>
> **Mast cells** are special white blood cells that produce histamine in response to an allergic reaction. They're involved in defending the body against foreign substances.

Take digestive enzymes

Take these with your lunch and evening meals. If you have multiple allergies, you might find that Polyzyme Forte from Biocare or Udo's Choice Digestive Enzyme Blend from Savant or Natural Woman helps to take the load of your digestive system by decreasing the amounts of undigested foods.

Do a regular detox

Easy-to-follow detox advice can be found in my book *The Complete Book of Food Combining*. I'm sorry that I don't have the space to cover detox here but following the dietary and other information in the chapter If You Do Nothing Else . . . (see page 250) should contribute considerably to cleaning up your diet and improving your digestion.

Get some herbal help

Certain herbal remedies can help to heal the gut in a number of ways. Both pau d'arco and oregano are anti-fungal. Barberry bark is anti-fungal as well as anti-parasitic, and may help liver function and to normalise bacteria, as well as having a beneficial effect on transit time. Goldenseal has natural anti-bacterial and anti-inflammatory properties and was used by Native Americans as a treatment for the digestive tract. Antioxidant milk thistle is famous for its liver-regenerating abilities. Freeze-dried garlic is anti-bacterial and anti-fungal, and inhibits the growth of *Candida albicans*. Olive leaf extract is effective at controlling *C. albicans,* bad bacteria and parasites, and so contributes to healing leaky gut syndrome.

Most of the supplement suppliers recommended in the Resource section (see page 323) can supply some or all of these products.

> For more information on specialist supplements, check out the Resource Directory (see pages 323–328).

> **A VERY IMPORTANT POINT**
>
> The dietary and lifestyle changes you need to get a grip on if you have leaky gut syndrome can seem daunting but are truly worth the effort. Left untreated, LGS can have serious long-term implications for the body's health and well-being.

Recommended reading

Leaky Gut Syndrome by Elizabeth Lipski.

Reducing the risk of leaky gut syndrome
KATHRYN'S TOP TEN TIPS

1. Avoid sugar, cow's milk, wheat cereals and bread, and any foods that contain yeast, white flour or artificial additives.

2. Read the chapter on candidiasis (see page 65).

3. Read the chapter on allergies (see page 115).

4. Read the chapter on intestinal parasites (see page 177).

5. Avoid alcohol, at least while you are getting well again.

6. Avoid cigarette smoke – yours and other people's.

7. Take a course of probiotics for at least three months.

8. Improve your digestion and reduce your toxic load – see If You Do Nothing Else . . . , page 250.

9. Take daily exercise and get plenty of fresh air.

10. Find yourself a good naturopath or nutrition-oriented practitioner who is familiar with the treatment of leaky gut syndrome, parasites and candida.

Check out the following for further information:
www.LeakyGut-subscribe@yahoogroups.com is a useful support group. When the home page opens, search Leaky Gut. It's easy to 'unsubscribe' at a later date by sending a blank e-mail to
LeakyGut-nomail@yahoogroups.com
Also worth visiting:
www.health-n-energy.com/leakygut.htm

20.

What's Up?
Ulcers

❦ Champions are pioneers, and pioneers get shot at. No support systems, no champions. No champions, no innovations. ❧

In Search of Excellence, Thomas J. Peters and Robert H. Waterman

> **Read this chapter if you have:**
>
> Acid reflux
> Indigestion
> Chest pain

Peptic ulcer is a general term for a sore that occurs when any part of the protective lining of the digestive tract is damaged. What happens is that stomach juices eat away at the gut lining, forming an ulcer. This could be in the stomach itself, in the upper part of the small intestine (the duodenum) or, more rarely, in the gullet (the oesophagus). A peptic ulcer in the stomach is therefore called a gastric ulcer (because it affects the gastric lining), a peptic ulcer in the duodenum is a duodenal ulcer and one in the oesophagus is an oesophageal ulcer.

The statistics I have – which are from the United States – show that one in ten people develop an ulcer, half a million new cases are diagnosed each year and more than a million people end up in hospital, often as a result of complications and/or late diagnosis. Left untreated, the lining of the stomach or intestines can be slowly destroyed, risking internal bleeding, vomiting of blood or blood in the stools. Even more serious is the possibility of perforation, where a hole in the membrane allows previously contained contents (partially digested food, for example) to spill into the abdominal cavity, causing contamination, infection, inflammation and life-threatening trauma. There is also evidence to show that untreated ulcers can lead to stomach cancer. Sorry to sound melodramatic, but I just want to convey the dangers that can occur if ulcers are ignored or incorrectly treated.

Until relatively recently, the accepted medical view was that ulcers were triggered mostly by stress (which disturbed the production of stomach acid), or by medications such as non-steroidal anti-inflammatory drugs (NSAIDs) or aspirin, and were probably aggravated further by rich, spicy or smoked foods, strong coffee, cigarettes and excess alcohol. Labelled the 'worry, hurry and curry culture', it was also believed that the rushed, stressed and ambitious A-type personality was more susceptible to ulcers than the slower, less-easily-flappable B-type personality. All these factors, it was reasoned, contributed to an excess production of stomach acid, which eroded the gastric lining.

Jargon buster

The word **peptic** comes from the enzyme pepsin, which digests protein.

Stress ulcers

There is no doubt whatsoever that persistent gnawing stress can eventually create the right conditions for a 'stress' ulcer to eat away at your stomach lining. So, too, can anxiety brought on by, for example, the worry of a stressful event such as a pending operation or a stay in hospital. It is also suggested that ulceration can be triggered by the stress of relationship problems, being trapped in a job or relationship and/or fear that we're not good enough – a sense of inadequacy that means we can't stomach who we are. An ulcer personality may be inclined to direct any aggression inwardly upon themselves. Outwardly self-assured and independent perfectionists may be developing an ulcer state of affairs by putting up a 'front' for their lack of confidence. Some research suggests that such types may benefit from *swallowing their pride* and admitting to their child-like reliance or need for maternal security. Page 304 has more information on stress and the digestion.

Beware

You could be at risk of contracting an ulcer if you:

- Smoke. Continued smoking can also prevent successful treatment.
- Drink alcohol to excess. This applies more specifically to the rarer oesophageal ulcer but can still be an issue in duodenal and stomach ulcers.
- Are under excessive and persistent stress.
- Take aspirin-based medication for the treatment of pain.
- Take non-steroidal anti-inflammatory drugs.
- Have either an excess or a deficiency of stomach acid.
- Eat a poor-quality diet.
- Hold on to your emotions.

Bacterial ulcers

Although any one – or all – of these conditions can increase the risk of ulcers, and might also hinder recovery, it's now known that by far the largest majority of ulcers are caused by a bacterium, *Helicobacter pyloridus* (usually written as *H. pylori*). It sets up home in the narrow space between the stomach lining and the mucous covering that tries to protect the stomach wall from damage, and aggravates the stomach into producing more acid, which then eats into the protective wall. Worryingly, it is now considered an even more prolific bug than salmonella!

The discovery of *H. pylori* has completely changed the way that ulcers are treated. The story behind this amazing discovery is fascinating.

The pylori story

In the mid-1980s, dedicated research by Australian doctors Barry Marshall and Robin Warren turned established practice on its head when they found a common bacterium called *Helicobacter pylori* nestling in the guts of a significant number of ulcer sufferers and dared to suggest that this bug could be *the actual cause* of ulcers. Marshall and Warren tried to interest the medical establishment in their discovery but were over-whelmed by a wall of apathy and indifference. Ulcers caused by bacteria? Don't be silly. Doctors have known for years that bacteria can't survive in stomach acid. (*H. pylori* actually has a very clever way of concealing iself so that it cannot easily be attacked and destroyed by hydrochloric acid, as are many other bacteria that find their way into the stomach.)

So firmly held was this belief that many medics didn't follow even the most basic hygiene rules, with the result that they unwittingly passed the bacteria from patient to patient during surgery and other invasive proced-ures. No one imagined for a moment that ulcers could be contagious! As Dr Marshall pointed out, no one believed tuberculosis or diphtheria were infectious a century earlier – or that it was possible to be a carrier without suffering symptoms.

The milk-based diet was, for many years, *the* remedy for ulcers, although it's now recognised as a poor protector against ulcer attack. Although this may soothe for a few seconds, once milk hits the stomach it stimulates the secretion of even more acid; it's akin to pouring pints of burning liquid over a raw wound, causing intense pain and further dam-age to the ulcerated area. Barbiturates, antacids, semi-comatose bed rest, stress-management techniques, psychodrama and, latterly, more sophis-ticated (and expensive) acid-suppressing drugs, have all come (and gone) as the treatments of choice. Now someone was suggesting that treating a bacteria was the answer.

Marshall and Warren were pioneers and they certainly attracted some flak. The two intrepid Aussies caused furore by suggesting that short-term treatment with the right kind of antibiotics (usually a cocktail of two dif-ferent ones with bismuth and, sometimes, antacids) could cure a very large percentage of cases. Early studies showed *H. pylori* to be evident in 73 per cent of stomach ulcers and 92 per cent of duodenal ulcers.

So convinced was Dr Marshall by his research (at Fremantle Hospital in Western Australia) that he used himself as the first guinea pig, swal-lowing a heavy suspension of the offending bacteria and giving himself an ulcer. Until he did this, the team couldn't be sure whether it was the bacterial infection that caused gastritis (inflammation and damage to the stomach lining) or if, perhaps, pre-existing inflammation allowed *H. pylori* to flourish. It's recorded that Dr Marshall's wife was, not surpris-ingly, extremely unhappy about his potentially dangerous experiment. But his dedication and commitment paid off and his antibiotic therapy worked, proving that it was, indeed, the bacteria that caused the ulcer.

> **Jargon buster**
>
> **Gastritis** occurs when the stomach lining itself has been damaged and becomes inflamed. Recurring or untreated gastritis can lead to gastric erosion, the first stage in the development of an ulcer where the mucous membrane has been eroded, exposing unprotected muscle tissue.

Dr (now Professor) Marshall's success was music to the ears of those who thought they would be on anti-ulcer medication for months or years – or for life!

When Dr Marshall presented his findings at an international medical conference, he was branded 'a little bit loony'. 'His trolley has come off the track' said one delegate. Since I found out about this, I've always had a burning ambition to ask that delegate what he thinks now! A colleague of Dr Marshall's wished he'd had a videotape of the gathering. He remembered that the audience of senior gastroenterologists 'couldn't take it' and stuck to their original views. Some even tried to blow the Marshall theory out of the water by carrying out their own studies – but ended up 'shooting themselves in the foot' by finding that the Australian had been right after all.

> **Scepticism and suspicion in the medical world**
>
> The BBC Horizon documentary *Ulcer Wars*, which did so much to highlight Dr Marshall's work, made the point that, despite several reports appearing in scientific and medical journals during the 1980s detailing the success of Dr Marshall's treatment, his discovery was ignored or dismissed for years. It's the way of the world that so many new discoveries, even if thoroughly tested and proven, can be held up for aeons by almost inevitable suspicion, scepticism and general slagging off procedures before they are acknowledged, agreed and approved for patient use.

Learning to keep an open mind

It can be positively healthy to be suspicious of anything new, but it is important to keep an open mind. In the eighteenth century, large doses of mercury were used to treat ulcers (the 'medicine' worked but the patients died!). Other health maxims of the time were that taking a bath or changing into clean clothing could be dangerous and that fresh vegetables were poisonous! But there were successes. Bismuth, an old-fashioned antiseptic astringent medicine, was also used (safely) and was 'rediscovered' by Dr Marshall.

So where do the bacteria come from?

Further research has established that *H. pylori* infection can be picked up in youth – sometimes as a result of poor or unhygienic living conditions and/or poor diet; or contracted from an infected carrier. Widespread infection is found most commonly in people who live in confined spaces and poor conditions where hygiene standards are low. The infection is present in saliva and in faeces. Once entrenched, the bug can be with you for good! Unless, of course, it's treated. Even if there are no apparent symptoms, it's possible for the person carrying the bacteria to pass them on to others who then develop the illness.

So strong is the possibility of the ulcer-causing infection being passed from one family member to another that, in some areas, screening programmes are being recommended to test and treat close friends and family. It isn't a question of catching the bug and contracting an immediate ulcer. *H. pylori* may not cause symptoms until the 'right' conditions prevail, such as other illnesses and lowered immunity.

The official view is that it's not possible to pick up the infection from animals. But I reserve judgement on this. If no one is yet sure how the bacteria get from the stomach of one *person* to another, and bacteria are rarely detected in human saliva, gastric juice or stools, I don't see how we can be so emphatic. It's known that animals do carry a similar bacterium and, until we know how *H. pylori* travels, it surely makes sense to practise good hygiene – to wash your hands thoroughly after working with or playing with animals and to never allow them to lick your mouth or face.

Who is at risk?

Ulcers can affect anyone, but some groups do seem more susceptible than others. They're slightly more common in men than in women and most likely to strike the mid-fifties upwards. It's suggested that people aged sixty-five and over may be more at risk as a result of poor living conditions during the Second World War. The prevalence of infection may also be increasing with age simply because of the ageing of the digestive system and changes in the natural production of digestive acids and enzymes.

In more detail . . .

Dr Marshall's experiments found that people infected with *H. pylori* can produce up to six times more acid than normal (the body's natural response to fight the infection), but also that in some patients the bacteria itself inhibit the production of stomach acid, increasing the likelihood of achlorhydria or hypochlorhydria – big words that mean non-existent or limited levels of acid.

The symptoms

The likely symptoms of a peptic ulcer are:

Gnawing, burning pain
Heartburn
Nausea
Vomiting
Diarrhoea
Pain in the shoulder blades
Pain associated with eating (stomach ulcers)
Pain that comes on two to four hours after food (duodenal ulcers)
Pain during the night

See your doctor

Don't delay in seeking medical advice if you experience any of the following:

- Persistent episodes of pain or burning in the stomach, chest or abdominal areas either after or between meals.

- If you have signs that could indicate internal bleeding such as:
  - Severe back pain that has no other explanation.

- Coughing or passing up anything that resembles dark coffee grounds.
- Passing stools that are very dark or black in colour.
- Unexplained tiredness, unusually pale skin, dizziness or weakness.

Medication for ulcers

H$_2$ blockers

Drugs called H$_2$ receptor-antagonists or H$_2$ blockers such as cimetidine or ranitidine can be effective in treating non-infectious ulcers. They work by blocking the production of histamine, a naturally produced chemical that triggers the secretion of stomach acid. This type of medication is sometimes also used in conjunction with antibiotic therapy for *H. pylori* infections.

Proton pump inhibitors

A stronger family of drugs known as proton pump inhibitors – omeprazole, lansoprazole and pantoprazole – act on the enzyme that triggers acid secretion and stops acid being produced altogether. Any one of these might be used with antibiotics to help eliminate *H. pylori*.

Both the H2 receptor-antagonists and proton pump inhibitors are still the treatments of choice for non-infectious ulcers, and they are indeed effective at healing peptic ulceration – but, unless antibiotics are prescribed simultaneously to eradicate the *H. pylori* bacteria, they may have limited long-term success. Dr Marshall himself discovered that it can be beneficial to use the acid-reducing drugs to relieve symptoms while the antibiotics go to work on the *H. pylori* perpetrator. However, there are cautions.

Using these types of drug to try to eradicate bacterial ulcers without antibiotic support is regarded as nothing more than a sticking-plaster approach in most cases. Not only are the ulcers extremely likely to recur, but also a greater danger lies in the fact that such medications can mask more serious disorders such as the early signs of oesophageal and stomach cancers. Now that these drugs are easily obtained without prescription, the American College of Gastroenterologists (representing some 5,000 specialists in more than thirty countries) expressed concern that as a result sufferers may delay seeing their doctors.

Antibiotics

Where the *H. pylori* bacteria are confirmed, a course of combined anti-biotics, sometimes taken together with one of the medications detailed above, is the most likely prescription. It may take up to three weeks for the bacteria to be eradicated.

Action plan for ulcers

You can reduce the risk of *H. pylori* returning (or bugging you in the first place) by following these simple steps. You may think that some of the suggestions are nannying or too extreme. You may belong to the school that says it's possible to be too fussy and that exposure to dirt and bugs helps to build resistance. *H. pylori* is not one to be ignored. Although its discovery has changed the way that doctors treat ulcers – instead of long-term medication, a short course of antibiotic therapy can clear up the condition – it is worth mentioning that it's all too easy to become reinfected, especially where there is lax hygiene. Most people harbouring the bacteria suffer no ill effects, but others will go on to develop gastritis and/or ulcers. One particularly virulent strain of the bacterium can cause damage severe enough to produce precancerous changes and could lead to stomach cancer.

So, if you think you may have an ulcer, here are my suggestions.

Your diet

Avoid milk products

This common allergen is still a suspect in the ulcer-aggravation department. And where an ulcer is already diagnosed continually drinking milk could slow down the healing process.

Consider the possibility of allergies to other foods

A diet that eliminates common food allergens has shown great promise in hastening healing and reducing the risk of recurrence.

For more information on how food allergies can affect digestion see page 115.

243

Enhance elimination of wastes

Up the amount of dietary fibre in your diet. Apart from vegetables, fruits, pulses and grains, include a tablespoon of crushed linseeds or psyllium powder daily. Page 271 has more information on dietary fibre.

Follow a basic supplement programme

This doesn't mean masses of different pills or potions but a sensible one-daily multi-vitamin and mineral and a gram of vitamin C.

Try raw cabbage juice and raw potato juice

Both are recommended by naturopaths for soothing gastritis, acid reflux and ulcers. It's believed not only that the nutrients in these raw foods help to soothe inflamed mucous membranes, but also that they may be able to neutralise acids in the system and rebalance mineral metabolism, thereby encouraging healing. They are not the most palatable remedies but there are ways to 'get them down' without too much grimacing. Liquidise fresh and tender raw cabbage leaves and a raw organic potato together with celery, carrot and apple. Make enough for three glasses of juice per day. Keep the juice refrigerated, and drink it before meals. It's also worth keeping the water from boiled potatoes and steamed cabbage and adding it to soups or juices. Also make soup with cabbage and a range of other vegetables. Use organic ingredients wherever possible.

Try soup made with carrot, parsnip and butternut squash

Rich in potassium and beta carotene, this is nourishing and comforting if your stomach is sore. Simply wash and chop the ingredients, cook until just tender, then blend into a smooth liquid.

Mash ripe bananas

They make a nutritious and easily digestible snack.

Invest in quality 'green' juice

It's a valuable top-up if you're not feeling like eating or are recovering from an ulcer or other illness. Packed with easily absorbable nutrients and simple to prepare, add it to soups or fruit juices. My favourites include Udo's Choice Beyond Greens from Natural Woman or Savant, Sweet Wheat from Natural Woman, Optimum Source Chlorella, Lifestream Spirulina or Pure Synergy, all from Xynergy Health, or Hawaiian Spirulina from The Naturopathic Health & Beauty Company.

In addition

- Avoid rich and fatty foods.

- Keep salt and coffee intake to sensible limits.

- Cut right back on sugar and don't eat too many sweets. Overindulgence on sweets can cause excess acid production.

- Eat a healthy diet rich in fresh fruits and vegetables.

- Buy organic whenever you can.

- Wash all fruits and vegetables thoroughly before use.

What else can you do?

Take certain supplements

Slippery elm is an ancient soother of mucous membranes and especially valuable if symptoms bother you at night. Take two slippery elm capsules or tablets (Biocare Gastroplex, Blackmores Slippery Elm or Bio-Health Slippery Elm) with water or make a drink with slippery elm powder (from a health food store) and organic soya milk, about half an hour before bed. Check labels and avoid wheat-based powders. Or try the Bioforce Silicea liquid that I mention on page 52. It brings immediate relief and encourages healing.

Some ulcer sufferers have reported that 20 millilitres of aloe vera juice taken twenty minutes before meals has helped ease their symptoms. However, take care to choose only the organic, cold-pressed juice. Try Biogenic Aloe Juice from Xynergy Health or Aloe Gold (Higher Nature).

Supplements containing a special kind of herbal liquorice (called DGL) can help to reduce inflammation and encourage healing of stomach and duodenal ulcers, and may also be useful for relieving heartburn. In at least one clinical trial, deglycyrrhizinised liquorice was as effective as anti-ulcer medication. Liquorice also has mild laxative properties. There has been some suggestion that excesses of liquorice might increase fluid retention and disturb potassium levels in the body, but this does not appear to apply to low doses. Although it hasn't been proven, if you use this valuable herb choose only those products containing DGL and make sure that your diet is high in potassium-rich fresh vegetables, salads and fruits. As an additional precaution, don't use liquorice if you have hypertension or are using diuretics or digoxin (digitalis).

Flavonoids, nutrients found in the pith, skin and bark of plants, and especially in dark-coloured berry fruits (cherries, black grapes, blackberries, bilberries, cranberries), are known to help ulcers. They dampen the production of histamine (which stimulates gastric acid) and also inhibit *H. pylori*. Antioxidant supplements are also a good source of concentrated flavonoids. Look out on the label for words such as pycnogenol or pine bark, green tea extract, grape seed extract, quercitin, rutin, hesperidin and ginkgo biloba. Brands I like include Solgar Advanced Antioxidant Formula or Advanced Proanthocyanadin Complex, Biocare Procydin and Viridian Pycnogenol with Grape Seed Extract.

Contrary to popular belief, some peptic ulcer sufferers may actually be deficient in hydrochloric acid and other digestive juices. Blackmores Celloid Mineral Chloride Compound can be a useful supplement for helping to regulate and balance digestive function.

Be scrupulous about hygiene

Inadequate hand washing, faecal contamination and careless food storage and preparation are three possible 'entry points' for *H. pylori*.

Take care when travelling

Be extra vigilant when travelling away from home, especially if you're visiting countries where there is poor hygiene, poor diet and untreated water supplies.

Clean your teeth regularly

Clean your teeth at least twice daily, disinfect your toothbrush at least once a week and see your dentist twice a year. Dental plaque can 'store' this bacterium, whence it passes into the unsuspecting stomach.

Purify your water

Filter your water – and change your filter cartridge regularly. Drink four to six glasses of freshly filtered water every day.

Watch the alcohol

Drink alcoholic drinks in moderation.

Keep equipment clean

Don't use anyone else's unwashed glasses, cups or eating utensils (even if you love 'em).

Don't smoke

Definitely don't smoke. It seems that heavy smokers are more likely to develop duodenal ulcers than people who don't smoke.

Watch the painkillers

Never take aspirin, and keep aspirin-based medication to a minimum. If you need painkillers, take occasional paracetamol instead of aspirin or non-steroidal anti-inflammatory drugs (NSAIDs) which, according to research, could be associated with increased risk of ulcers 'at all dosage levels; no conventionally used prophylactic aspirin regimen [being] free of the risk of peptic ulcer complications'. The combination of NSAIDs and cigarettes seems especially harmful; the drug itself causing the ulcer and the smoking stimulating the gastric acid to make symptoms worse.

Take probiotics

Follow a course of probiotics at least once a year and always after antibiotics (see page 294). Maintaining a healthy balance of intestinal flora not only strengthens immunity but, research shows, also inhibits the growth of *H. pylori*. In some countries, doctors will prescribe probiotics routinely; in the UK (at the time of writing), this therapy is not available on prescription and is rarely offered, but it's still worth asking your GP. Be aware that not all probiotic products contain the quantities of bacteria claimed on the label. Go for quality brands such as Biocare, Higher Nature, Viridian, Solgar or Pharma Nord.

For more information on probiotics see page 294.

Avoid stress

Do whatever you can to protect your system from stress. It's well known that stress can aggravate illness; digestive disorders are no exception. Ask anyone with an ulcer and it's likely they'll admit to feeling more pain and discomfort when they are under stress than when they are not. It's impossible to avoid tension and anxiety but, by looking after yourself properly, you can provide your body with the nutritional and other support which it needs to cope with stressful situations. A good diet, the right supplements and daily destressing relaxation techniques, such as positive visualisations, progressive relaxation, deep breathing and sensible levels of exercise, are all important buttresses against the negative effects of stress.

Get tested

If you have a family history of ulcers or have anyone in your household who is – or has been – a sufferer, ask your GP to test you for *H. pylori*, too.

If you have already received antibiotic treatment for *H. pylori* but your ulcer or gastritis has come back, ask for repeat tests to be carried out. Relapse rates may be higher if the wrong (or the wrong combination of) antibiotics were used and did not completely eradicate the bacteria. Dr Marshall found that one kind of antibiotic in isolation was not sufficient to deal with the infection.

VERY IMPORTANT POINT
Peptic ulcers can be extremely dangerous if not treated effectively. Therefore anyone with a suspected or diagnoised ulcer should be monitored by a qualified doctor. If you're not sure whether this applies to you but you suffer frequently with burning sensation or pain in the chest, stomach or abdomen, then do see your GP. If you have been taking any kind of acid-suppressing medication or anti-ulcer drugs for more than a

few weeks but are still suffering symptoms, go back to your doctor and ask for further tests or a second opinion.

Long-term use of these drugs is not to be recommended. Apart from a number of known side-effects, it is likely that symptoms of more serious illness might be masked and therefore missed. If no one seems to be listening, don't be afraid to be pushy. It's possible to have a low-level infection and/or small ulcers that have not been spotted in routine tests, so if you've a persistent or recurring problem with dyspepsia or gastritis, it might still be beneficial for you to go the antibiotic route, even though your tests for the bacteria have proved negative. It's been estimated that those infected with *H. pylori* (who remain untreated) could be twice as likely to suffer from heart disease and six times more likely to develop stomach cancer. So, if in doubt, get yourself checked out.

Reducing the risk of ulcers

KATHRYN'S TOP TEN TIPS

1. Don't smoke.

2. Drink alcohol in moderation.

3. Cut right back on sugary, fatty foods.

4. Don't take aspirin on an empty stomach.

5. Keep NSAID and aspirin-based medicines to a minimum.

6. Deal with stress.

7. Eat a diet rich in fresh produce and wholefoods.

8. Avoid cow's milk.

9. Make personal hygiene a priority.

10. Improve your digestion (see page 251).

21.

If You Do Nothing Else...

❝ Don't tell your friends about your indigestion. 'How are you' is a greeting, not a question. ❞

A Poet's Proverbs: Of Tact, Arthur Guiterman, 1924

I provide you with a lot of information in this book. I know you won't get around to using it all. With the best will in the world, and however keen anyone might be to get well, sometimes it seems as if we all have so much else to do that health takes a back seat. I don't have to tell you how essential it is to give yourself some space, to be a priority in your own life, to stop putting everyone else first and take care of number one for a change. But I know you won't. Well, you might do it for a while but then you'll forget and drift back to your old ways – until the symptoms that made you buy this book give you a bit of a kick up the backside and, hopefully, you'll stop and think that maybe you should look after yourself a bit better than you do.

So, this chapter is for you. I hope you'll read it, read it again and promise yourself that you will, definitely, from now on, introduce at least some of it into your daily routine. And *please* read it if your digestion ain't so great or if you have *any* of the conditions detailed in the What's Up? section of the book. All the recommendations that follow are gentle pointers to take the strain off your overworked gut and to nurture it to work more efficiently. For the benefit of your long-term health. From me to you. The chapter is divided into five parts.

1. Swap that for this

2. Lifestyle and dietary hints

3. Recognise potential gut-wrenchers

4. Eat more of the superfoods

5. Soothing remedies

1. Swap that for this

Below is the expanded and updated version of my 'swap box', which is aimed at improving the actual quality of your food choices. The column on the left-hand side contains foods that most of us would buy without thinking. The column on the right has the healthier options. If you make just one or two changes at a time over the next few weeks, you'll not only be giving your body more nourishment, but should also be avoiding many of the ingredients that are known to disturb the digestion.

Instead of this	**Go for this**
Deep-fried food.	Stir-fried, steamed, grilled food; food that has been cooked in a wok or casserole.
Food cooked in a chip pan or deep fryer.	Food cooked in a steamer, skillet or wok.
Processed cooking oils. Most mass-produced polyunsaturated oils – sunflower, corn, etc. – are heat treated, stripped of nutrients and processed using chemical solvents.	*For cooking* Cold-pressed canola oil or extra-virgin olive oil. From health food stores and some supermarkets. *For dressings, drizzling onto cooked vegetables, jacket potato or salads, adding to soups or pasta, or blending into juices or smoothies* Cold-pressed nut or seeds oils such as flax, pumpkin seed, safflower, sesame, sunflower, walnut, avocado or grape seed. Add two or three teaspoons daily of cold-pressed oil to your diet. Available from health food stores or check Resource Directory (see page 323). Don't forget to store all cold-pressed nut and seed oils in the refrigerator. It's OK to cook using extra-virgin olive oil, but remember that other cold-pressed oils are damaged if they are heated.

Instead of this	Go for this
Margarine or low-fat spread.	Organic butter (from most supermarkets), or non-hydrogenated spread such as Vitaquell or Biona (from health food stores), or pumpkin seed butter (from some independent health food stores and by mail from Higher Nature). Alternatively keep your olive oil in the fridge. It thickens and becomes 'spreadable'.
Crisps and peanuts.	Almonds, Brazil nuts, hazelnuts, macadamia nuts, pecan nuts, walnuts, sunflower seeds, pumpkin seeds.
Chips.	Sliced potatoes sautéed in extra-virgin olive oil (or for occasional convenience buy organic ready-cut chips).
Mashed potatoes.	Organic jacket spuds.
Sweets and cakes.	Health food stores have a great range of sweet treats. Look out for wholegrain cereal bars (avoid those that list sugar near the top of the ingredients), halva, natural liquorice, dried fruits, fresh fruits and Spirolight Fruit & Nut Bar (Xynergy Health).
Sprinkling sugar or artificial sweeteners.	Best-quality honey (such as Comvita Manuka), real maple syrup, blackstrap molasses (rich in iron and kind to the bowels) and organic brown sugar.
Rich desserts.	Soaked dried fruit compote. Organic ice cream; soya ice cream – one of my favourites is Berrydales. Or for a nourishing dessert, mash a banana with half a carton of sheep's or goat's milk yoghurt and a teaspoon of Comvita Manuka honey.
Chocolate.	Sensible amounts of organic chocolate (it's delicious).
Packaged fruit juices, especially orange juice. Processed juices are not recommended. Many of them are reconstituted and contain colourings, sugar and acids.	Organic apple or grape juice, Organic Biona Cranberry juice. Consider investing in a juicer machine and making fruit and vegetable juices from fresh produce at home. Add one of the green juice powders to your fruit and vegetable juices for extra nourishment. Page 244 has information on this.

Instead of this	Go for this
Coffee, tea and cola drinks.	Savoury beverages, Miso soup, vegetable soup, water, fresh fruit juice, vegetable juice, herbal fruit teas, Bambu or dandelion coffee substitute. If you use ordinary tea, why not choose the organic option?
Battery or barn-raised poultry and eggs.	Organic/free-range poultry and eggs.
Wheat-based or sugar-coated cereal.	Oat porridge, gluten-free muesli, rice puffs or millet flakes. Your health food store is the place for non-wheat cereals.
Cow's milk.	Soya milk, oat milk, almond milk or Rice Dream – or very small amounts of organic cow's milk.
Cow's milk cheeses and yoghurts.	Sheep's or goat's milk cheeses and yoghurts, avaliable from some supermarkets and health food stores. St Helen's Farm, Delamere Dairy, Raven's Oak Dairy and Woodlands Park Dairy all specialise in goat's and/or sheep's milk, butter, cheeses and yoghurts. Website and other contact information for theese companies can be found in the Resource Directory (pages 323–328). If you do use cow's milk cheeses, *please* choose organic varieties.
Ordinary mass-produced bread.	Yeast-free soda bread, pumpernickel, rye bread, rice cakes, oat cakes, oat biscuits, Matzos, pittas – or invest in a bread-making machine and make your own bread using organic ingredients. It's so easy, you'll wonder why you never did it before. Check your health food store and supermarket for organic wheat-free/gluten-free breads, crispbreads, cereals, flours, pastas, pizza and pancake mixes. See Resource Directory (page 323) for stockist information.
Non-organic beef or pork.	Fresh fish, lean lamb, free-range organic poultry.
Convenience meals and takeaways. Did you know that the UK consumes 1.9 million ready-made meals – on average six times more per year than any other European country?	Prepare meals from your own fresh basic ingredients so that you know what goes into them. They don't need to be elaborate or take long to prepare. Simple meals are often the best.

Instead of this	Go for this
Canned vegetables. Most canned foods are high in salt or sugar, or both.	Fresh and frozen vegetables. For those who resolutely refuse to like fresh vegetables, try blending some into soups. Adding Viridian Blue Food Blend or Udo's Choice Beyond Greens is a fast-track way of getting concentrated vegetables into reluctant relatives!
Salt, ketchup, vinegar.	Try Herbamare and Trocomare flavoured salts, and Kelpamare liquid seasoning. All are available from Bioforce. Also try Seagreens Table Condiment from Xynergy Health, and organic yeast-free stock cubes, available from health food stores and some supermarkets. Fresh herbs and dried herbs, including coriander, fennel, rosemary, mint, parsley, sage and dill, are all rich in nutrients and helpful to the digestion. Health food stores stock a wide range of additive-free seasonings. If kids insist on ketchup, choose an organic brand.
Foods full of additives.	Foods that aren't! Always check food labels and say no to E numbers, artificial colours, preservatives, flavours, emulsifiers, stabilisers, fillers, modified starch and any chemical-sounding names.
Same old stuff? Most of our meals are based on only a handful of foods, in particular wheat and dairy products.	Introduce more variety. It's the easiest way to get more nourishment into your diet. Buy a wider selection of fresh fruits and vegetables, choose Asian dishes, shop at the Italian or French counter. Be more adventurous with your menus.

2. Lifestyle and dietary hints

Even with the above improvements, there's not much point in following a healthy diet if your system isn't able to digest it properly. This section is full of ideas to help your gut get back into gear. Don't try to cover all the points at once. Go slowly. Introduce one or two new changes every week.

Get up a few minutes earlier

Do this each morning to give yourself time to 'potter around' and have breakfast. This isn't as difficult as you might think, and once in the habit, you'll really appreciate the extra space. The old adage: 'Breakfast like a king, lunch like a prince and dine like a pauper' really does make good digestive sense. If you honestly cannot face food first thing in the morning, eat some fresh fruits and yoghurt or drink fresh fruit juice or vegetable juice (which is filling and nourishing) as soon as you feel able to. Avoid running on empty until lunchtime.

Never eat on the hoof

Make every effort to sit down to regular meals and remain seated for ten minutes after you've finished eating. Give yourself time to unwind. A relaxed stomach will digest far more efficiently than a tense one.

Food combine

There is absolutely no doubt that, for many people, avoiding concentrated protein/starch combinations really can improve digestion and absorption, and that for many people it does certainly improve bowel function. My kind of food combining also removes common allergens from the diet and increases the intake of fruits, vegetables and fibre. Even used as a short-term emergency measure, taking more care with food combinations can take the strain off the system and hasten recovery. See page 283 for more.

Eat fruit separately

Don't eat fruit at the same time as proteins and starches. In other words, eat them between meals or as entrées before other food. Mixing fruit with other foods is one of the single most common causes of indigestion. People often blame the fruit when the problem is actually caused by the unwise combination. This tip was consistently voted one of the very best preventive measures by my students. If you're an irritable bowel syndrome sufferer, check out my note about fruit in the food-combining section (see page 284).

Learn about food

Learn about the food you buy and the food you eat:

- Read a fabulous book by Joanna Blythman called *The Food We Eat* and her follow-up *The Food Our Children Eat*.

- Read everything you can that is published by the independent watchdog the Food Commission, in particular their excellent publication the *Food Magazine*. Find out more from www.foodcomm.org.uk.

- I also highly recommend *Diet For A New America* by John Robbins.

Go organic

Choose the organic options whenever possible. Organically grown foods are known to contain more nourishment than the commercially raised equivalents. It's also interesting that some people who appear to suffer adverse reactions to non-organic produce can cope comfortably with non-sprayed alternatives.

That doesn't mean you should give up fresh fruits and vegetables if organics are unavailable. Some stores still put excessive premiums on organic produce, pushing prices out of reach of many consumers. However, the Soil Association (see page 326) can provide valuable information on organic food supplies in your area that shouldn't cost the earth!

In the meantime, always wash all fruits and vegetables before use to remove as much pesticide residue, dirt and bacteria as possible. If fruits feel waxy or look perfectly unblemished, the chances are they've been sprayed, so it's best to discard the peel. Let's hope that, eventually, we'll see the introduction of 'P' numbers enabling shoppers to check which pesticides, herbicides, fungicides and preservatives have been used on their potential purchases, and so to make an informed choice.

Eat little and often

It's better for your digestion and your bowels than going for long periods without food, resorting to rubbish snacks and then filling up with a large meal once a day. Even the most nourishing of foods cannot be digested properly if you overload your system.

> **Beware**
> It's worth knowing that very hot or very cold foods can cause indigestion. Could this be because stomachs were invented before cookers or refrigerators?

Go easy on the fibre

If you're taking the advice to increase your fibre intake (see page 271), begin with small amounts. Too much too soon could cause discomfort.

Loosen your clothes

Tights, girdles, belts, skin-hugging jeans or loads of Lycra make it more difficult for your digestive system to work efficiently – it's rather like not being able to breathe properly. On particularly painful or bloated days, go for the extra-baggy and loose look. Comfort is king when you're not feeling well.

Keep warm

Keep your hands, legs and feet warm. Chilly extremities can make bowel discomfort worse.

Take care when eating out

This may sound obvious, but it really is far healthier to avoid rich meals and keep food simple. For example, choose jacket potatoes instead of chips, pass on the sauce and ask for extra vegetables or a side salad. Don't 'experiment' with unfamiliar or potentially troublemaking foods when you are eating away from home or have an important 'daren't miss it' day ahead. Play safe.

Avoid rushing meals

Don't gallop from entrée to main course to dessert. Pace yourself and leave a little time between courses. Chat, read a few pages, people watch, look out of the window . . .

Did you know?
Ginger is one of the best remedies if you're feeling sick.
A tiny splash of gin in a glass of hot water is an old remedy for settling the stomach.
Fennel tea can help relieve gas.

Check your posture

Don't forget what I said about posture (see page 172). Leaning forwards or sitting in a slouched position can cause considerable discomfort – so check your posture. Abdominal cramps, heartburn and hiatus hernia may be relieved by improved posture. Deep-breathing exercises are recommended for anyone suffering from digestive distress. When the chest muscles become cramped and tight, it's easy to mistake the discomfort for digestive or heart problems.

Realign your spine

If chronic indigestion persists and your GP can find nothing wrong, consider seeing a chiropractor or osteopath for a course of treatment. Lesions of the thoracic spine can alter the nerve and blood supply to the gut, aggravating poor digestion.

Reduce your toxic overload

Do this by:

- Restricting your use of household chemicals. Most of them are not necessary.

- Buying environmentally friendly products, especially washing-up liquids and loo cleaners. Try the new E-Cloth system – reusable cloths that clean glass, stainless steel, worktops, ceramic and all other hard surfaces using just water. Stockist details are included in the Resource Directory (see page 323).

- Choosing organic hand-wash and skin-care products (Green People, Neal's Yard, Jurlique) natural herbal or mineral toothpaste (Green

People, Bioforce, Blackmores) and deodorant (Pitrok, Crystal Spring, Green People). These brands are my personal favourites – further details are in the Resource Directory – but independent health food stores should also have a wide range of different makes to choose from.

- Filtering your drinking water.

- Keeping aluminium out of your life. It can cause gas and distention. That includes avoiding aluminium cookware, including aluminium pans, other utensils and foil, unfiltered water and packets of dried food. Be wary of proprietary indigestion remedies. Many of them contain aluminium. So do some toothpastes.

- Becoming an avid label reader and making every effort to avoid packaged foods that contain artificial colourings, flavourings or preservatives.

Also check my notes on pages 122, 126 and 128 on organics and food additives. These changes aren't difficult or expensive to introduce and are especially important if you're suffering from candidiasis, allergies, irritable bowel syndrome or leaky gut syndrome.

Take regular exercise

Coupled to a healthy diet, it's essential for improving bowel function and is believed to lower the risk of serious bowel disorders by as much as 40 per cent! If you're housebound or for any reason unable to walk or take other more vigorous exercise, even simple movements such as deep breathing, massage and arm stretches can make a difference. People who are able to practise t'ai chi or yoga report that bowel behaviour improves as their muscles become stronger and stress levels reduce.

Whatever exercise you go for, don't overdo it – and avoid vigorous exercise immediately after a meal. During and immediately after eating, the heart works harder to divert blood supply from the muscles to the abdominal area to aid digestion. Research demonstrates that rushing around too soon after eating can cause severe cramps and strain to the heart. Those with angina or other heart/circulatory disorders should take special care.

Helpful hint

Upset tum? To help settle a sore, acid stomach, mix two tablespoons of sheeps milk yoghurt with one tablespoon of plain, cooked, white basmati rice. Take in small spoonfuls and chew each mouthful thoroughly.

Get rid of gas

Exercise can relieve gas. If you feel bloated or are in pain from gas pressure, go for a gentle walk or stretch, then sit down, bring your knees up to your chin and stretch again. Alternatively, lie down on the bed, bring your knees to your chest and rock gently from side to side and then backwards and forwards. Do this somewhere privately – gas may be expelled! Another way to relieve discomfort is to take a warm bath. Massaging the abdomen each night (see page 78) improves muscle tone and helps to relieve wind pain.

Give up smoking

If you smoke, make every possible effort to give it up. Cigarettes have a hugely detrimental effect on the digestive system and on the bowels. They cause the stomach to over-produce acid and are implicated in ulcers. And apart from the known links to lung cancer and heart disease, it seems that the old fag can also increase the risk of far more serious gut disorders such as Crohn's disease and ulcerative colitis.

Did you know?

Every cigarette shortens a smoker's life by fourteen minutes. That means you lose nearly five hours a day for every packet of twenty, and that for every five packs, life gets shorter by nearly a whole day!

3. Recognise potential gut wrenchers

If you're trying to get your digestion into shape or are suffering from any kind of bowel disorder, the following foods may be best avoided, at least until you are feeling much better.

- Wheat-based foods such as:
  Wheat bran
  Breakfast cereals
  Bread
  Crackers
  Biscuits
  Cakes
  Pastries and pies
  Quiche and pizza bases.

- Cow's milk.

- Corn (maize).

- Corn sugar/syrup.

- Rice syrup.

- Anything that contains 'modified starch': check labels, especially on low-fat and other packaged foods. Modified starch is often used as a fat-replacing bulking agent.

- Yeast.

- Sugar and sugary foods.

- Beef and pork (lean lamb is usually well tolerated).

- Artificial additives, including colourings, artificial flavours, preservatives and sweeteners. Sorbitol seems particularly problematic, so do check labels.

- Very hot or very cold foods (remember that stomachs were invented before cookers and refrigerators).

- Oranges and orange juice.

- Eggs, especially if you have gall-bladder problems.

Watch your coffee intake

Replace one or two cups of coffee per day with two glasses of water. Try green teas, fruit teas and coffee substitutes. If IBS-linked diarrhoea is a problem, coffee may be best avoided altogether.

> **Tomatoes and Onions**
> These are generally considered to be very good for you, but they do seem to increase the production of stomach acids in some people so go easy on them if you suffer from acid reflux.

Be aware of potential irritants

This is especially the case if you have an ultra-sensitive system or suffer from hiatus hernia, reflux, ulcers, touchy tum or temperamental bowel. Salt, pepper, curry, spices, chocolate, soda pop and alcohol (and coffee) are worth avoiding for a while, or at least cutting down on.

> **Rhubarb and Plums**
> Rhubarb and plums can gripe a sensitive stomach, especially if made into pies.

Stay off the sugar

Keep off all sugar and sugary foods if you possibly can. Apart from all the bad things you already know about sugar, it's not good news for the digestion either. Sugar not only feeds any yeasts that are in the gut, but its absorption also uses up a lot of body energy and heaps of nutrients.

Avoid cigarettes

Do whatever you can to avoid cigarette smoke, especially around mealtimes. It's a real gut wrencher and, in addition to its many other unhealthy attributes, is known to aggravate the production of stomach acid.

4. Eat more of the superfoods

These are the good gut foods that you should include regularly in your new diet:

- Psyllium husks.

- Linseeds.

- All kinds of fresh fruits – aim for two to three pieces daily between meals. Also good are all kinds of dried fruits (great with fresh sunflower and pumpkin seeds as a snack or with Brazil nuts or almonds – unless you are allergic to nuts). Apples, bananas, berry fruits, fresh or dried figs, papaya, prunes, pears and raisins are especially valuable. **Fruit intake may need to be reduced during the early stages of candida treatment. Consult your practitioner for further advice.**

- All kinds of fresh vegetables and beans, including broccoli, cabbage, Brussels sprouts, chickpeas, kidney beans, lentils, cauliflower, asparagus, globe and Jerusalem artichokes, sweet potatoes, pumpkin/squash, carrots, turnips, swede, leeks and onions.

- Fresh garlic – if you don't eat it or don't like the taste of it in your food, take a daily garlic capsule with your main meal.

- Organic potatoes in their jackets and cold cooked potatoes.

- Vegetable soups and juices. Fresh carrot juice is particularly recommended.

- Cereal foods: oat bran and oat biscuits, oat bran porridge (easiest to digest when made with water), rye bread and rye crackers, brown rice, rice cakes, rice pasta, buckwheat, millet and wheat-free muesli. Important note: for most people, oats and rye are an excellent source of fibre that is kinder to the gut than wheat. But be aware that they do also contain some gluten – although much less than wheat does. Health food stores stock good ranges of gluten-free foods including muesli, pasta, flour and so on. Yeast-free products are also available.

- Cold-pressed oils such as extra-virgin olive oil or pumpkin seed oil.

- Yoghurt, made from sheep's or goat's milk and unflavoured.

- Blackstrap molasses.

- Manuka honey.

Fresh is best

Consume groceries well within the use-by date. Don't store canned food once it has been opened. Use it up. (Very fresh sauerkraut and very fresh yoghurt can be extremely healthy. Aged, poorly stored products can be just the opposite.)

Use a fridge/freezer thermometer

Check storage temperatures for your foods regularly. If you're unsure whether your fridge or freezer is cold enough, turn it down a notch to a cooler temperature anyway.

Try to avoid reheating food

If you do need to use cooked leftovers at the next meal, make sure they're refrigerated and then reheated thoroughly. Never reheat ready-made meals or takeaways.

Figs

Fresh and dried figs are a wonderful source of dietary fibre, and also provide calcium, magnesium, carotene, potassium and iron. Said to be good for the digestion and one of the very best remedies for a sluggish bowel, they're a healthy sweet alternative to biscuits, cakes and chocolate. In the United Kingdom, fresh green figs are usually in the shops before Christmas and are available right through to July; Turkish black figs are generally available from late summer to autumn. Both types can be eaten with the skin. Figs can seem expensive but they're cheap compared to bars of chocolate. Chop fresh or dried figs into a tub of sheep's milk yoghurt and add a sprinkling of pumpkin and sunflower seeds for a really delicious and nutritious snack or dessert.

Tips on using vegetables

If you find it difficult to digest vegetables (for instance Brussels sprouts, broccoli and cabbage), or know someone who refuses to 'eat their greens', then cook the vegetables for a little longer and mash them before serving. While they may not contain as much nourishment as raw or lightly cooked vegetables, they will still be good for you. Not everyone has a taste for crispy al dente.

If certain vegetables still give you gas or discomfort, don't be too keen to blame the food itself. It may be that your digestive system is under-functioning and unable to break foods down efficiently. Or it could be that the food in question only causes pain or bloating if it's eaten in the wrong combinations. Here's what to do: leave the current troublemakers out of your diet for now. Put as much of the information in this book into practice as you can. When your symptoms have reduced and you're feeling better, reintroduce – one at a time – any foods that previously upset you. Thereafter avoid them only if they still cause you discomfort.

Drink any water left over from cooking vegetables – it's full of nourishment and can be soothing to a sore stomach, peptic ulcer or irritable bowel. If drinking it 'straight' doesn't appeal (although it's amazing how our attitudes to such things change when we're suddenly unwell), chill the liquid in the refrigerator and mix with home-prepared vegetable juice or use in soup or a sauce. Don't allow your kitchen sink to become 'the best fed mouth in the house'!

Spicy food – a help or a hindrance?

It's worth mentioning that although many people complain that foods such as chillies or curries tend to aggravate their digestion and irritate their bowel, there is some evidence that spicy food can also be protective. Research carried out in Singapore shows that chilli stimulates mucus secretion, which gives increased protection to the stomach lining, thereby reducing the risk of upset. If spices spike you, it's highly likely you know it already. So, probably the best advice is to avoid them if they give you grief and to enjoy them in moderation if they don't!

5. Soothing remedies

Drink aloe vera juice

Add it to your daily fluid intake. This pleasant drink can be refreshing, cleansing and calming, and seems particularly helpful for irritable bowel syndrome, ulcers, hiatus hernia, acid reflux, nausea, candidiasis, indigestion and stomach upsets; it's comforting, too, after a heavy night out! Aloe vera eases inflammation and may help to promote healthy gut flora.

To drink aloe vera, take 40 millilitres first thing in the morning, once or twice during the day – between meals – and again before bedtime. As a soothing douche for piles, anal irritation, thrush or cystitis, dilute 20 millilitres of aloe vera juice in 250 millilitres of water (approximately four teaspoons in half a pint). Replace the bottle cap securely, keep the juice in the refrigerator and use it up within a month. Buy only cold-pressed aloe juice such as Xynergy's Biogenic Aloe or Aloe Gold from Higher Nature (see page 323). Juices of a lesser quality may not be effective and can taste extremely bitter.

Use a herbal indigestion remedy

Choose a herbal alternative indigestion remedy for the first-aid cupboard. Meadowsweet has soothing antacid properties, relieves distention and wind, helps combat infection and is one of the best remedies for heartburn, gastritis and the soreness of hiatus hernia. Sometimes combined with other plant remedies or with charcoal, it's available in tablets from health food stores. Activated charcoal not only absorbs gas but also helps to bind and eject toxins from the system. Try Potters Acidosis Tablets or KiwiHerb Meadowsweet & Aniseed. Slippery elm (in capsules or powder) is soothing for all the mucous membranes that line the digestive tract, calming inflammation and irritation throughout the body. It is especially helpful in cases of indigestion, reflux, acidity, ulcers, irritable bowel syndrome, hiatus hernia, diarrhoea, catarrhal conditions and cystitis. Try Blackmores Slippery Elm, or ask in your local health food store. Or try Bioforce Silicea (see page 52).

Rest your digestion

If you're striken with a stomach upset, the best course of action is to rest the digestion for twenty-four hours. Drink plenty of water and take acidophilus – two capsules every four hours (see page 294). Small quantities of freshly cooked brown rice and organic grated carrots or carrot juice are healing and cleansing.

Take vitamin C every day

It's been my experience that a low-acid or 'buffered' vitamin C taken before meals not only helps to improve regularity but may also reduce inflammation and the risk of infection. Blackmores, Bioforce, Biocare, Viridian, Higher Nature and Solgar all have good vitamin C products. Avoid those large vitamin C tablets that you dissolve in water; they can be very acidic and may upset a dodgy digestion. Irritable bowel syndrome sufferers should take vitamin C after a meal.

Take linseeds or psyllium husks

Add them to your daily fibre intake. Both these fibres are gentle, soothing and loosening. Begin with one teaspoon of seeds or husks per day and increase by one teaspoon per day (to a maximum of five teaspoons – three is usually about right) until you achieve a soft and easy bowel movement. Always take linseeds or psyllium with a large glass of water. Mix psyllium husks into water or juice and drink immediately. Blend into juices or smoothies or follow the suggestions in the chapter on dietary fibre (see page 271). Brands to consider: Linusit Gold from health food stores and some supermarkets; Cold Milled Flax Seeds or Colofibre (psyllium) from Higher Nature; Udo's Choice Beyond Greens (Savant or Natural Woman) or Psyllium Husk from Solgar.

Go for some digestive enzymes

Take a course of digestive enzymes, one with lunch and one with your evening meal. You'll remember from my description of the small intestine (see page 17) how incomplete digestion of proteins can lead to a number of potentially obstinate health problems including overgrowth of yeasts, decaying of untouched food, allergies, parasites and a greater risk of infection and inflammation. A month or two of good-quality enzyme supplements can take the strain off an overworked digestion, improving the breakdown of starches, fats and proteins, and increasing absorption of vital nourishment. I would recommend Biocare Digestaid, an old favourite with a good track record, Viridian Digestive Aid, Udo's Choice Digestive Enzyme Blend (available from Natural Woman or Savant), Solgar Vegetarian Digestive Aid or G&G Digestive Complex.

Note that digestive enzymes may not be suitable if you have gastritis, acid reflux or ulcers. Check with your doctor or nutrition practitioner before taking them.

Detox yourself

Following a regular but simple two-day detox is a great way to rest the digestion. There is no need to go to any kind of extreme. Just avoid all foods except vegetables, fruits and fresh, plain sheep's or goat's milk yoghurt. Ignore normal mealtimes but don't allow yourself to feel empty. Anytime you are hungry, eat fruits, salad foods or lightly cooked vegetables. Drink plenty of water, soups, vegetable juices and herb teas – but don't eat fruits at the same time as vegetables.

> There's more information, including recipes, on the two-day detox in my best-selling book *The Complete Book of Food Combining*, available from bookshops, or through **www.amazon.co.uk.**

VERY IMPORTANT POINT

If none of these things improves your condition, see a naturopath or doctor who is familiar with nutritional treatment and is able to test for allergies and to isolate any underlying digestive disorders. When you ring for an appointment, find out if they are willing to get together for a ten-minute 'meet and chat' before you commit yourself to a full consultation. If travelling distances make this difficult, at least ask to speak personally to them on the telephone. If they're too busy for you before treatment, they are unlikely to be there for you during or after it!

Good gut health

KATHRYN'S TOP TWENTY TIPS

1. Use the 'swap box' (see page 251) to improve the variety and quality of your diet. In particular, find alternatives to wheat-based cereals, bread and cow's milk. If you use cow's milk, keep it to an absolute minimum and only buy organic.

2. Remember that meat makes the gut work really hard so consider introducing more fresh fish and/or vegetarian options. If you do eat beef, lamb or pork (or chicken), choose organic. In fact, choose the organic options for all food wherever they're available and when you can afford them.

3. Keep sugar and sugary foods to a minimum.

4. If you drink alcohol, be sensible about intake and don't drink on an empty stomach. Avoid beer, lager, sweet sherry and liqueurs. Of all the alcoholic beverages, they seem to aggravate symptoms most.

5. Become an avid label reader and don't buy foods that are loaded with additives.

6. Eat fruits first – at the beginning of a meal.

7. Drink more water, especially between meals (see liquid news, page 289)

8. Eat more dietary fibre and take psyllium husks or linseeds every day (see fibre tips, page 271).

9. Allocate a couple of days each month to rest your digestion, and give your liver a holiday by eating only salads, fresh vegetables and juices. *The Complete Book of Food Combining* (see opposite) has more information on detox and there are several dedicated detox books available to help you, including *The Detox Cook* by Louisa J. Walters, *Detox Plan* by Jane Alexander and *The Liver Detox* Plan by Xandria Williams.

10. Take probiotics for three months every year and always after antibiotics. Buy the best you can afford. Page 294 has more information.

11. Take a multi-vitamin/mineral supplement five days a week and 500–1,000 mg vitamin C every day. Choose top-quality products such as those by Biocare, Blackmores, Bioforce, Higher Nature, Solgar and Viridian.

12. Sit down to meals.

13. Chew your food slowly and thoroughly.

14. Breathe more deeply and steadily and learn to relax (see digestion and stress, page 304).

15. Make every effort to avoid cigarette smoke – yours and other people's.

16. Take more exercise but don't make strenuous movements right after eating.

17. Massage your abdomen daily.

18. If you have recurring or persistent digestive or bowel problems, talk to your GP or practice nurse.

19. **Remember to enjoy what you eat** Include a wide variety of different foods, be moderate and don't go to extremes, but don't fall into the trap of thinking that if it tastes awful it must be healthy or that if it tastes great you should feel guilty.

20. **Never forget that your health is your wealth.**

22.

Essential Extras: Fibre Tips

6 It's said that medical men in China were once so revered that patients thought it adequate treatment merely to swallow the paper on which the prescription was written. 9

Anon

An ancient equivalent, perhaps, of the breakfast box containing more nourishment than the cereal?

What is dietary fibre?

Dietary fibre is found only in foods of plant origin: cereals and grains, fruits, legumes or pulses, nuts, seeds and vegetables, and comes from the part of the fruit, vegetable or cereal that we can't digest. Fruit juices and vegetable juices are low in fibre. Meat, fish, milk, eggs, butter and cheese have zero dietary fibre.

Why is fibre so important?

Dietary fibre isn't essential only to those with bowel disorders. It plays an important role in the prevention and treatment of disease and is a vital part of general health care. Fibre acts like a natural broom, helping to sweep wastes along the tube, preventing a build-up and keeping the walls of the colon free of stale faeces. This is just one of the ways that a high-fibre diet composed of unrefined grains, fresh fruits and vegetables helps prevent such conditions as constipation and diverticular disease, and encourages healthy intestinal function.

> **Did you know?**
> In the large intestine, fibre is partially broken down by bacterial fermenta-
> tion which produces nutrients called essential fatty acids that are crucial
> for a healthy bowel.

High-fibre stools are two to three times as bulky as those lacking fibre. By
adding bulk to the diet, more fluid is absorbed – think about taking a dry
sponge and pushing it down into a bowl of water. Once soaked, wastes
are softer, 'cleaner' (less mucusy) and easier to pass. And transit time is
speeded up from a sluggish thirty-six hours or more down to an average
of between twelve and twenty-four hours. As a result, the gut is healthier because the mushy stuff doesn't get a chance to hang around and go
off! In fact, fibre actually helps to clean up the encrusted walls and stimulate local circulation. Although a large proportion of the water content
is reabsorbed as the mush works its way through each section of the large
intestine, sufficient moisture should remain at the end of the passage to
make for comfortable defaecation.

Low-fibre diets make for tacky, mucus-laden faeces that stick to the
colon wall. Abnormal bacteria build up, producing harmful carcinogenic
substances. Elimination is slow and poor, taking three times as long – or
longer – to make the journey. This delay encourages excess water absorption, leaving dense stools that require much greater pressure and force to
reach the exit. This also puts undue strain on the colon walls, increasing
the risk of those out-pouchings we were talking about in the chapter on
diverticulitis (see page 105). Some wastes never reach the outside world,
getting jammed up against the wall and into the pouches where they
putrefy (go off), then solidify and stick. Well, I did warn you this book
wasn't all lace tablecloths and bone-china teacups.

Is all fibre the same?

There are two main types of fibre: soluble and insoluble. All plants have
some of both kinds, but some plants have more soluble or more insoluble. These terms can seem confusing but all they really mean is that the
fibre either dissolves in water (soluble) or doesn't (insoluble). One type
of fibre is not better than another. They do different tasks and both are
essential for good health.

Insoluble fibre

This provides a plant with its structure. The insoluble fibre in our diet passes undigested into the large intestine and provides bulk to the stools. The reason it's sometimes called 'roughage' is because it is actually 'rough'. The most familiar source of the insoluble stuff is wheat bran, but it's also found in other wholegrain foods, some vegetables and fruit skins. This is the kind of 'roughage' that is famous for keeping bowels regular. It may also reduce the risk of some types of cancer.

Soluble fibre

Soluble fibre – vegetable gums and lignins – is predominant in legumes (pulses), vegetables, fruits, oats, barley, rye, seeds and psyllium husks. In the digestive process it's broken down into a jelly-like mass which, in contrast to the rough stuff we looked at above, is soft and smooth. It helps to shift hardened faecal matter in the lining of the colon wall and may have an important role in reducing blood cholesterol. Soluble fibre can help lower LDL (bad) cholesterol, and it slows down the rate that glucose (sugar) enters the blood and so is believed to be especially important for diabetics.

Resistant starch

Another type of fibre that has only been talked about since comparatively recently is something called resistant starch, a type of starch that 'resists'

Did you know?

Fibre is known to have at least six main functions:

1. Improving transit time and assisting the movement of wastes through the gut;
2. Balancing the levels of blood glucose; foods high in fibre are digested more slowly. which puts the brakes on sugar absorption.
3. Stabilising cholesterol and reducing the risk of heart disease.
4. Helping to protect against haemorrhoids, varicose veins, diverticular disease, gallstones, kidney disease and constipation.
5. Reducing the build-up of toxins, yeast and pathogenic bacteria.
6. Binding and deactivating carcinogens, helping to reduce the risk of colon cancer.

digestion. It's found in cereals, fruits and vegetables. It seems that some starchy foods develop more resistant starchy components after they've been cooked. One example is cold cooked potato. Resistant starch is fermented in the gut by bacteria in much the same way that other fibres are. When this happens, it produces those essential fatty acids I mentioned earlier (see page 272), which are believed to be important in reducing the risk of colon cancer. In response to this finding, scientists and food technologists have developed a type of corn, known as Hi-maize, which is high in resistant starch. It's what they call a 'functional food' and is now included in some mass-produced breads and other packaged goods in an effort to increase the fibre content of foods that are usually low in fibre.

The disease risks (particularly for heart disease and bowel cancer) for people who eat low-fibre diets, and can't or won't eat wholegrain bread or vegetables, are extremely high. It seems Hi-maize is being hailed as a real health benefit because it can be incorporated into convenience foods without affecting lightness and quality. This is how some brands of white bread have suddenly become 'high fibre' without looking or tasting any different. It's a way of getting fibre into otherwise non-fibrous food – you could say without the consumer realising its there. It's said to improve colonic health, increase the bulk of stools and slow the absorption of sugars. I think I'd rather get my dietary fibre from natural sources.

A word about wheat

Many people are perplexed by their condition because they do eat plenty of fibre. But more often than not, it's wheat fibre. I've been going against the wheat grain for years, writing articles about seemingly ubiquitous, less-than-helpful cereals that resemble brown string and sawdust. Renegade that I am, I've been suggesting we don't use wheat.

Unfortunately, for some people, plain old wheat bran can sometimes be more of an irritation than a help. If you're wheat-sensitive, it's a bit like expecting something with all the smoothness and charm of a ball of Velcro to pass snag-free down the length of an 8-metre (28-foot) nylon stocking. My experience has certainly been that wheat bran seems to irritate, aggravate and inflame, especially in conditions such as leaky gut syndrome and irritable bowel syndrome. I sometimes wonder if this 'intestinal mayhem' existed in such epidemic proportions before the fibre faddists persuaded us that it was a good idea to eat the equivalent of at least one equestrian nosebag every day and call it breakfast cereal.

Recently, there have been several reports in highly regarded journals that confirm that wheat bran may not be as helpful as the conventional medical establishment once suggested. Perhaps sensitivity to wheat rules out any benefits its fibre might have bestowed? Whatever the reason, can I suggest this: if you have no problem with wheat-based foods in general or with wheat bran in particular, then by all means include it in your diet and gain the benefits it has to offer – but don't eat it to excess. If all kinds of wheat upset you, find other fibres that might suit you better, such as oats, linseeds, whole rye, brown rice and psyllium. If you go with the bran option, don't overdo it. Apart from the problems with sensitivity and excess flatulence that I talked about earlier, bran can bind up essential minerals like iron. If you have irritable bowel syndrome, avoid wheat bran totally.

Beware

If you're sensitive to wheat and dairy foods, bran cereal drowned in cow's milk is a double-whammy; two common irritants that end up in the same bowl. Instead, try porridge made with water, or oat bran cereal or wheat-free muesli with organic soya milk. Check the labels on cereal packets. Some contain 'hidden' wheat.

Did you know?

The wheat that is used in so many of our food products is mass-produced, hybridised bread wheat, quite different from original natural wheat grains. We don't always realise that it's everywhere in the diet. But when you add the wheat biscuits, the sandwich bread, the cake, pastry, pie crust, pasta, pizza base, quiche base, sauce, gravy and a multitude of processed, packeted and tinned convenience foods – all containing wheat – to a day that began with breakfast bran and toast, overload becomes an understatement. Not surprisingly, the body can become sensitive to a particular food if it is consumed in such large amounts.

It's interesting that the old wheat grains such as spelt and kamut (which are now much more widely available via health food stores and delicatessens than they once were) are often well tolerated by people who react violently to modern bread wheat; they may even prove to be suitable where there is gluten sensitivity. It seems that the structure of the gluten in spelt differs from that in common bread wheat. So it's worth testing small amounts for tolerance.

VERY IMPORTANT POINT

High-fibre diets should never be given to children under five years of age or to elderly people. An infant gut will not have matured sufficiently to cope with excess amounts of fibre. In later life, narrowing of the large intestine, reduced mobility, lack of fluid intake, poor diet or poor digestion can reduce the body's ability to cope with large amounts of fibre, which can cause compaction, blockage, severe pain and even death. If a very young or elderly person is constipated, consult a doctor, health visitor or practice nurse before attempting to give laxatives or additional dietary fibre.

Helpful hint

One kind of very gentle fibre which can be used for young and old is a superior water-soluble type that glories in the fabulous name of fructo-oligosaccharide. (try F.O.S. for short). F.O.S. encourages healthy growth of an important friendly flora called Bifidobacteria. F.O.S. is available from Biocare and is also included in Viridian's very good Fibre Complex. See Resource Directory page 323. There's more about probiotics on page 294.

How to boost your intake

Here are a few tips for boosting your fibre intake:

- Steer clear of coarse wheat bran. Instead, introduce oats, brown rice, brown pasta, pulses, plenty of fresh fruits and vegetables and organic jacket potatoes into your diet (can I suggest you don't eat the skins on non-organic spuds).

- Use plenty of peas, beans and lentils. Try organic baked beans as a filling snack. Stock up the store cupboard with canned pulses and chuck them into all kinds of dishes. Add mixed pulses to soups, casseroles and salads. Make hummus paste with chickpeas, garlic and olive oil. Include foods from the list of fibre providers on page 80.

Caution: if you have gallstones or gall-bladder problems, eat pulses (legumes) only in small amounts. There's more on this on page 144.

- Drink plenty of fluid. It helps your body to use fibre safely.

- Promise yourself that you'll eat at least two pieces of fresh fruit every day.

- Add a side salad and an extra vegetable to your main meal.

- Every time you shop, try a different vegetable or fruit. And don't forget that, although frozen fruits and vegetables are usually peeled, they still have some dietary fibre and are good standbys when fresh equivalents are unavailable.

- Instead of cakes, chocolates, biscuits and crisps (chips in America), snack on fibre-rich foods such as seeds, nuts, carrots, apples and dried fruits.

Did you know?
Chewing every mouthful really thoroughly at every meal helps your body to break down dietary fibre and digest food more efficiently.

- Use oat bran to make smooth porridge. Mix it with water, not with milk, and sweeten it with a teaspoon of New Zealand Manuka honey. It's available from health food stores or check the Resource Directory (see page 325) for stockists.

- Eat a wide variety of foods to ensure that you get the best possible range of nutrients and the right amount of fibre.

Helpful hint
If, for you, beans means fartz, then improve digestibility by soaking dried beans for at least eighteen hours. This helps to remove a large percentage of the starches that give off all that gas. Throw away the soaking water and cook in fresh water, skimming away the 'flatulence foam' and changing the water at least once during the cooking process. If you short cut with cans, then rinse the contents thoroughly through a sieve until all the foamy bubbles disappear.

- Snack on mixed dried fruits, and sunflower and pumpkin seeds. Unless you're allergic to them, unblanched almonds, walnuts and Brazil nuts are excellent sources of fibre.

- Soaked dried fruits such as apricots, prunes and figs provide fabulous fibre, plenty of nutrients and a sweet treat.

VERY IMPORTANT POINT

Don't add lots of fibrous foods to your diet all at once. A gradual increase gives your body the chance to adjust. Introduce too much too quickly and you're bound to get bloated and gassy.

- Include flaxseeds – also known as linseeds – regularly in your diet. Not only rich in both omega 3 and omega 6 fatty acids, they're also what herbalists call mucilageous (slippery) and demulcent (soothing). These qualities make linseeds one of the most gentle and effective bulking agents. Start with a teaspoon per day, either first thing before breakfast or after your evening meal. Best way to take them?

1. Either pop the seeds into your mouth from the spoon and drink at least half a tumbler of water, letting the liquid wash the seeds down.
2. Or cover the seeds with filtered water, leave them in the fridge for a couple of hours, then stir them into yoghurt.

Do this for one week, then increase your intake to two teaspoons daily. After a further seven days, increase again to three teaspoons, making sure you increase your water intake accordingly. Then stay on this dose for as long as you like.

Choose plain organic golden linseed such as Linusit Gold – available from health food stores and some supermarkets – or one of the excellent organic flax products from Higher Nature. I really enjoy the Green People Organic Omega 3&6, which I sprinkle on to yoghurt, cereals and salads, and into juices. Always keep flaxseeds in the refrigerator to protect them from rancidity. Seeds that cost less or are sold loose may not be the good value they seem. Exposed to light and air, the nutritious oils in the seeds will almost certainly have degraded. Never take linseeds without increasing your fluid intake.

- Linoforce, a Bioforce product, is also based on linseeds, but it has other ingredients, including senna, and can be especially helpful if bowels are really sluggish. I have positive feedback to the effect that this product is the one to choose in the weeks following surgery for haemorrhoids (see page 159). A little Linoforce goes a long way, so try half a teaspoon per day to begin with and increase by half a teaspoons until an easy bowel movement is achieved. Never exceed the stated dose and don't take it at the same time as other laxative preparations.

- Psyllium seeds and husks have high levels of soluble fibre, which expands and takes on a gelatine-like appearance when in contact with water. This bulks the stools, reducing their density and easing the passage of waste through the large colon. The gentle behaviour of psyllium stimulates normal peristaltic activity without causing cramping or griping. Psyllium also helps to break down the build-up of mucus and undigested proteins in the gut, making it a valuable natural, drug-free, internal cleanser that encourages the removal of putrefactive toxins from the intestines.

  Psyllium's adaptogenic and regulatory action also makes it a useful supplement for the treatment of diarrhoea, constipation, diverticulitis, haemorrhoids and irritable bowel syndrome. Higher Nature's psyllium-based Colofibre and G&G Psyllium are both available by mail order. Solgar Psyllium Husk should be in your local independent health food store. Contact details are in the Resource Directory (see page 323). Take psyllium with lots of water.

- If you travel a lot and have to rely on other people to prepare your meals, or if your fibre intake takes a dive while you're on holiday, consider packing your own high-fibre cereal and dried fruits (such as apricots and figs).

- 'Portable' fibre supplements can be a helpful standby if, for any reason, you're not able to follow a naturally fibrous diet, for instance if you're away from home or if someone else is in control of your meal choices. Some hotel menus are, let's face it, decidedly lacking in the healthy high fibre department. Fibre supplements are not habit forming and don't contain chemical laxatives. They can be a useful addition to the diet if fresh vegetables or wholegrains are not in evidence. Do keep in mind, though, that supplements usually contain only one or maybe two kinds of fibre and therefore don't give you the variety you'd get from a fibrous diet. It's also worth knowing that it takes around four or five fibre-filled capsules to provide the same amount of fibre as one apple or one banana. In addition, a fibre supplement doesn't provide the vitamins and minerals – or, for that matter, the taste – that you get from food. So use them wisely and in moderation.

Good fibre supplements include Bio-Fibre from Pharma Nord, Colon Care capsules from Biocare, Blackmores Herbal Colon Care powder, Higher Nature's Colofibre, Arkopharma Ispagula or Fibre Complex with F.O.S. from Viridian.

For more information on where to find specialist supplements and food products check out the Resource Directory on pages 323–328.

How much is enough?

Official recommendations vary around the world, but a good guide is between 25 and 30 grams of dietary fibre per day. Don't worry about calculating or weighing exact amounts. You'll get enough daily fibre if you ensure that, whatever you decide to eat, two-thirds of your meals are made up of fruits, vegetables or grains.

Which foods for fibre?

There are many good sources of dietary fibre that can be relied upon to 'do their thing'. Here are just a few:

Almonds	Cannellini beans
Apples	Carrots
Apricots – fresh or dried	Celery
Asparagus	Coconut
Bananas	Cold, cooked potatoes
Barley	Courgettes
Beetroot	Dried fruits
Black eye peas	Figs – fresh or dried
Blackberries	Jacket potatoes
Blueberries	Lentils
Broccoli	Lima beans
Brown rice	Linseeds
Brussels sprouts	Nuts
Cabbage	Oats

Peaches	Raspberries
Pears	Sesame seeds
Peas	Snow peas (sugar snap peas)
Potatoes in skins	Spinach
Prunes	Sultanas
Pulses	Sunflower seeds
Pumpkin seeds	Sweet potatoes
Raisins	Whole rye

Check the astonishing difference between the fibre content of these foods. A quick glance at the graph below shows you how easy it is to increase your daily fibre quota just by swapping white rice for brown rice, white pasta for wholemeal pasta, peeled or mashed spuds for jacket

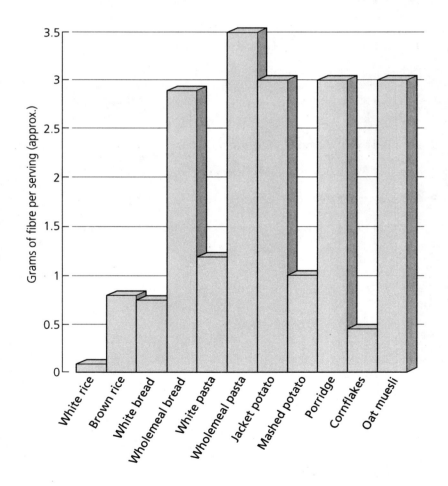

potatoes, refined breakfast cereal for oats or muesli. If you add fresh fruits, salad foods, and a wide variety of vegetables, beans and seeds, you'll certainly be up there with the best fibre providers.

Improving your intake of dietary fibre

KATHRYN'S TOP TEN TIPS

1. Increase your fibre intake slowly over a period of a few weeks.

2. Begin by adding one extra piece of fruit and one extra vegetable every day.

3. The next week, try wholemeal bread, rice cakes or rye crackers instead of white bread.

4. Try oat porridge or muesli instead of bran cereal or flakes.

5. Drink a glass of water before each meal.

6. Add new and different vegetables and fruits to your shopping basket each week.

7. Eat dried fruits instead of sweets and chocolate.

8. Take a dessertspoon of linseeds every day with a glass of water or juice.

9. Buy organic potatoes (new or old) and eat them with their skins.

10. Sit down to your meals and chew every mouthful thoroughly.

23.

Essential Extras:
Food Combining

> 6 To eat is human, to digest divine. 9
> Mark Twain, 1853–1910. Also attributed to Charles Copeland, 1860–1952

This section is about food combining for farts ... and for easing constipation, bloating, indigestion and acidity, and improving transit time.

Remember our journey through the digestive system (see page 10) and
how we looked at transit time (see page 29)? Remember that proteins take
longer to digest than starches, which take longer than vegetables, which
take longer than fruits? And fats take longer than anything? For some
people, especially those who don't digest their food fully, mixing all these
foods together at one meal doesn't work too well at all. Foods that need
to stay for longer in the stomach may hold on to other foods that would
prefer to get away. Or sometimes, fast-transit foods can push slower foods
through to the next stage of digestion before they're ready.

This is where food combining comes in. Careful combining means that
foods get the chance to be digested more fully. As transit time improves,
what we've eaten is less likely to ferment, give off gas or cause bloating.

Helpful hint
Try food combining if you suffer from:

Acid reflux	Candidiasis	Diverticulitis	Haemorrhoids
Bloating	Constipation	Dyspepsia	Hiatus hernia

If you haven't tried food combining in the past or gave up on it because you found it too complicated, then I do implore you to read more about my very simple system of food combining. It sounds covetous to say 'my system' because this dietary concept has been around for many years and has been written about most excellently by many other writers. However, my own particular recommendations, which are borne out of a number of years in clinical practice, and of conversations with and feedback from patients, are different in a number of respects from other methods. In particular, my system has only two main 'maxims' and is entirely flexible. One of the reasons I set out to make sure of this is because I believe that when someone isn't feeling well, the last thing they need is a diet full of rules and regulations or dogma. I'm sure this was a right decision to make. The feedback, for example, on *The Complete Book of Food Combining*, confirms that people do find it extremely easy to follow. I've therefore included some very basic steps here in the hope that you will find them helpful, too.

Just in case you have never come across food combining before, I should tell you that it really involves nothing more than not mixing protein foods with starchy foods at the same meal. It doesn't mean that you give up proteins or starches – simply that you don't eat them together.

There are only two rules you need to follow:

1. Eat fruits at the beginning of a meal or between meals, but not in the middle nor as a dessert. In other words, eat fruits on an empty stomach.
2. Don't combine concentrated proteins with concentrated starches at the same meal.

1. Introducing the 'fruit rule': here are some suggestions

Drink fruit juice (diluted one-third water to two-thirds juice) first thing in the morning as soon as you get up, saving breakfast until after you're washed and dressed;
or
Instead of your usual breakfast, eat two pieces of fresh fruit;
or
Enjoy a banana or a pear as a mid-morning snack;

or
Snack on a bunch of grapes or a glass of apple juice during the afternoon;
or
Instead of eating fruit salad as a dessert after your evening meal, enjoy it at the beginning of the meal.

2. Not combining starchy foods with proteins

If you're not familiar with food combining, this can seem a strange suggestion but it does make a lot of sense. It does not mean that you need to eat everything separately.

- Proteins combine well with vegetables and salads.

- Starches (carbohydrates) also combine well with vegetables and salads.

Proteins – that means meat, poultry, eggs, cheese, fish and soya – need an acidic environment to begin their digestion.

Starches – that's pasta, bread, potatoes, and all the grains including rice, oats and wheat – require alkaline conditions (non-acidic) to be fully digested.

Why the mix matters

As soon as proteins arrive in the stomach, acids are produced to begin the process of protein digestion. But starches don't like to be mixed with acid. Their digestion is triggered by the enzymes from saliva, which of course provides alkaline conditions, not acid ones. It's a fact of life that starch digestion will come to a complete stop if there is acid in the stomach. So if you eat protein and starch together in the form of meat and potatoes, fish and chips, chicken and rice or pasta and cheese, acid will be secreted to meet the protein, but all those starch-digesting enzymes from your saliva will be deactivated and nothing else will happen to that starch until it reaches the small intestine.

People who are strong and healthy and are not struggling to cope with a troublesome digestive or bowel disorder will find that they can eat mixed meals without noticing any symptoms. They may not fully digest the meals but will still absorb sufficient nourishment from them to

285

maintain good health. But when the system is struggling the results can be very different. It's possible that, if you find food combining helpful, you may not need to follow it all the time. Even a limited amount of sensible food combining can help considerably to ease digestive discomfort and encourage the healing process.

Here's the deal

Begin by food combining one meal each day, preferably your evening meal. If you find that your symptoms improve, increase your food-combined meals to two per day. If you achieve a good combining regimen for five days out of every seven or for two meals out of every three, you should gain considerable benefit.

Here's how the major proteins and starches fit into food combining:

PROTEINS

OK with salad foods

OK with vegetables (but not potatoes, yams and corn)

OK with oils, spreading fats, nuts, seeds and dressings

Not OK with starches or fruit

Major proteins include:

Beef	Game	Soya products
Cheese	Lamb	Textured vegetable protein (TVP)
Chicken	Pork	Tofu/beancurd
Eggs	Quorn	Turkey
Fish	Soya milk	

STARCHES

OK with salad foods

OK with potatoes, yams and corn

OK with oils, spreading fats, nuts, seeds and dressings

Not OK with proteins and fruit

Major starchy foods include:

All kinds of grains:	All kinds of pasta:	All kinds of bread:
Barley	Buckwheat pasta	Ciabatta
Buckwheat (kasha)	Durum semolina	Crackers
Bulgur	Kamut	Matzos
Couscous	Spelt	Oat Biscuits
Millet		Pitta bread
Oats	Corn	Pumpernickel
Quinoa	Potatoes	Rice cakes
Rice	Sweet potatoes	Rolls
Rye	Yams	Rye bread
Semolina		Rye crackers
Wheat	Sweet biscuits	Soda bread
Wild rice	Cakes	Wraps (tortillas)
All types of lentils, peas and beans except soya	Cereals Porridge Muesli	All types of flour

IBS and food combining

This is an interesting situation. On the one hand, I have seen a considerable number of patients who tell me that food combining has provided a major improvement to their irritable bowel syndrome (IBS) symptoms and that when they *don't* follow the two rules (see above), the condition flares up and they don't feel so well. On the other hand, I have talked to a number of people with IBS who say that while they find not mixing proteins and starches can be very helpful, the particular rule of eating fruits on an empty stomach doesn't suit them at all and can make their symptoms worse.

All illnesses have their individual differences, and where one person may have one set of symptoms, another may experience entirely different reactions. IBS seems, almost more than any other condition that I have come across, to be a very personal illness where things that apply to one sufferer often don't affect someone else. As in the case of the anomaly about sugar intake that I described in the section on IBS (see page 202), it's useless to suggest that everyone with IBS should fit a rigid pattern of symptoms or reactions. All I can say is that if you are unfortunate enough to suffer from this distressing and stressful condition, you may like to try my food-combining recommendations and see if you note any improvements. If there are no changes, or if you think you feel worse, then of course you should not consider food combining as part of your treatment.

The following letter, e-mailed to my publisher, was so kind and generous. This excerpt demonstrates that a simplified version of food combining can be just as effective as a complicated routine.

I would be grateful if you would pass on my gratitude to Kathryn for writing . . . *The Complete Book of Food Combining.* The work she put into it must have been overwhelming yet it is simply and caringly written with the author's sincerity clear to all. I have been a convert for several months . . . and feeling much better . . . since becoming a combiner. I [had been] confused about many points [and] Kathryn has cleared all these up and provided much on which to ponder. The recipes are so easy and . . . a joy to prepare. Please tell Kathryn how much I enjoyed and learned from her book.

Mrs R.K., South Wales

24.

Essential Extras: Liquid News

<blockquote>
Medicine is a collection of uncertain prescriptions, the results of which . . . are more fatal that useful to mankind. Water, air and cleanliness are the chief articles in my pharmacopoeia.

Napoleon Bonaparte (it didn't help his haemmorhoids though!)
</blockquote>

An important point that is often missed when we talk about dietary fibre is the need to increase our intake of liquids – preferably water. Many people 'forget' to drink simply because they don't feel thirsty, and yet to work efficiently and safely dietary fibre demands fluid. I've noticed dehydration and lack of water intake to be extremely common, especially in older patients and in children. Boosting fluids is an important adjunct to relieving the discomfort of conditions such as constipation and diverticulitis, but is also essential for good general health. Sometimes doing nothing else but upping the daily fluid quota is enough to cure constipation.

But how much is enough?

Many of the diet and health books that we read suggest anything from six to eight or perhaps more glasses of water per day. But this can seem excessive, especially if you think it means drinking large amounts all at once, leaving you feeling bloated and what a colleague of mine calls 'kind of swilly'.

One of the easiest ways to check your intake is by knowing what quantity the cups and glasses in your house actually hold. Most large glasses and large mugs hold half a pint (around 250 millilitres) of liquid. Average teacups, small mugs and small tumblers take about a third of a pint (just under 200 millilitres). If you aim for ten of the smaller measures each day, giving you 2 litres or just over 3 pints, you'll be doing well. Men of average build and moderate activity levels should go for twelve of the smaller cups, making nearer 2½ litres or 4 pints each day.

This doesn't have to be an exact science, so don't go mad on the measuring. Include as much water in this total as you can but don't forget that soup, tea and juices also count. And bear in mind that your needs will be less if you eat plenty of fresh vegetables, salad foods and fresh fruits. You know what happens if you liquidise fresh produce into juices? Well, your body makes liquid from those foods in just the same way.

You may feel you need more than this if you work out, run or are involved in sports, or if you sweat a lot.

VERY IMPORTANT POINT

Still not sure how much you should be drinking? A rough but useful guide is to count five large glasses of water each day *in addition to other fluids*.

Rather than take in a full glass of water all at once, it can help to 'spread it around'. Always carry water with you, in your bag or in the car. Leave filled glasses on your desk and around the house, in the kitchen, the bathroom, the bedroom. Take a mouthful each time you're reminded. You'll be surprised how quickly they are emptied. Drinking a glass of water a few minutes before each meal is another way to up your daily quota.

If you don't enjoy the taste of tap water, filter it. Bottled water is an option if you're away from home or travelling, but it's expensive. The cost of a jug and a regular change of filter is small compared to how much you would spend on the equivalent amount of bottled water.

Drinks with meals?

Too much liquid with food can dilute the digestive juices so that they become less effective. Not enough can leave food too dry. A small glass of water, especially if you need to swallow medication, supplements or digestive enzymes, is about right. If you take a glass of wine with a meal, you should still include the glass of water.

> ### Estimating if you're drinking enough
> You can tell if you're getting enough water by how many times you empty your bladder each day and by the colour of your urine. Six to eight visits per day is fine. Fewer than six could suggest that you might be a bit dehydrated, especially if your urine is dark yellow or strong smelling instead of pale yellow and inoffensive in smell. The exception to this colour rule is if you are taking supplements. The first urine of the day can also be darker simply because no fluid has been taken into the body during the night. Vitamins such as B2 (riboflavin) provide a strong orange colour to urine, but this is quite normal and healthy. Foods that might colour up your pee are beetroot, carrots and dark green leafy vegetables.

What about different types of drink?

- **Enjoy wine in moderation** Take comfort from the fact that a glass of good cheer (red or white) can help the digestion. Excess alcohol is likely to have the opposite effect!

- **Tea and coffee** taken with food can disturb digestion. Enjoy them, but drink them between meals, not with or immediately after food.

- **Avoid carbonated drinks** unless you find them particularly helpful in bringing up gas. If so, keep them for 'medicinal' use only. For most people, all that extra carbon dioxide only makes their digestive discomfort worse.

- **Avoid bottled orange juice** It isn't always the health booster that you might think. Not only does it seem to cause stomach pain in some people, but quite a lot of it isn't as natural, real or pure as the packaging might lead you to believe. Some orange drinks are only kept in supermarket chiller cabinets to make you think they're perishable. In reality, they're so full of additives that they'd survive at room temperature for years. Check the label on the brand you usually buy.

Did you know?

For every glass of orange juice, 220 litres (48 gallons) of water is used in the production process and to irrigate the orange crop. Hardly a sustainable use of such a precious resource, especially in some of the most water-scarce areas of the world.

Helpful hint

Improve the taste and remove a substantial quantity of chemicals by filtering your tap water. Chlorinated water can cause quite severe indigestion. I've known people who have spent months trying to isolate the particular food that they thought was upsetting their digestion only to discover, eventually, that it was the chlorine or the fluoride in their tap water that was the cause.

Recommended Reading

If your water supply is fluoridated or is likely to be so in the future, I would very strongly recommend that you read *Fluoride: Drinking Ourselves To Death?* by Barry Groves.

Make sure of your fluid intake

KATHRYN'S TOP TEN TIPS

1. Drink a glass of water when you first wake up in the morning.

2. Drink another glass of water ten minutes before your midday and evening meals.

3. Leave bottles or glasses of water or juice near to your workspace and around your home; take a mouthful each time you see them.

4. Always carry water in the car, in your bike bag or holder and anytime you're travelling.

5. Keep coffee and alcohol intakes to sensible limits; the're both dehydrating.

6. Eat more fresh fruits.

7. Add a side salad and an extra vegetable to your main meal.

8. Every time you visit the bathroom, freshen up your hands and face and then take a drink of water.

9. Exchange at least one cup of coffee per day for a coffee substitute (dandelion 'coffee' or Bioforce Bambu), or apple or cranberry juice.

10. Have soup regularly, as a starter to a meal or as a snack.

25.

Essential Extras: Probiotics

❝ There are more microbes per person than the entire population of the world. Imagine that. Per person. This means that if the time scale is diminished in proportion to that of space, it would be quite possible for the whole story of Greece and Rome to be played out between farts. ❞

The Old Country, Alan Bennett, 1978

This section explains the role of intestinal flora, describes bacterial overgrowth and how it damages our intestines and advises on replenishing the good guys.

So what else turns you on?

The gastrointestinal tract is home to vast quantities of bacteria – over 500 different types – weighing in at anything up to a couple of kilos. Some are harmful, some are friendly. In a healthy gut, there will be a higher ratio of good bacteria keeping the not-so-good bacteria under control. But where the good guys are in short supply, movement of wastes slows right down (that's because they're in charge of peristalsis), and rubbish backs up and goes off, providing a delicious and consistent food supply for the bad bugs. They feed, multiply, blow bubbles, spit toxins, make you fart and make you smell. Strong, unpleasant odours emanating from any-where in or on the body – for instance from the feet, the mouth, under the arms, or the groin, or from gas emissions – are the results of multiplying and decomposing bacteria. Waste products are no exception.

Did you know?
More than half the weight of the average low-fibre turd is made up of not-so-friendly bacteria, and most of the rest of it consists of undigested food (what a waste).

When bacteria or yeasts get at our food, not only do they cause it all to ferment and produce loads of gas, but also in the process they manufacture all kinds of other unpleasant substances, in particular vasoactive amines. These compounds upset the blood supply to the muscles that support the intestinal tract, increasing the permeability (the number of holes) of the gut, causing abdominal pain and slowing down the transit time of food.

Symptoms of bacterial overgrowth
The major symptoms of bacterial overgrowth in the intestines are similar to those of inadequate digestive enzymes or low levels of stomach acid:

Indigestion	Bloating
Burping and belching	Flatus/gas
Strong-smelling faeces	Borborygmi (abdominal rumbling)

Reducing bacterial overgrowth

There are several ways to prevent bacterial overgrowth and to restore the balance.

- **Avoid sugar** – it uses up nourishment and feeds the bacteria.

- **Eat more fibre** to improve the transit time of food through the gut.

- **Repopulate with probiotics** to restore the levels of friendly bacteria.

- **Regularly massage the abdomen,** in particular the ileo-caecal valve (see also page 78). This valve is the 'doorway' between the large and the small intestine. If it loses its tone and become lazy, bacteria from the large intestine can flow back into the small intestine, increasing the population of bad bugs.

- **Strengthen immunity, deal with food allergies, address that stress.** In other words, check out any malfunction that affects the production of an antibody known as secretory IgA. This antibody protects mucous membranes from damage by bacteria, so anything that reduces it, such as adverse reactions to food, poor immune function or excessive and persistent stress, is contributing to bacterial overgrowth.

- **Take digestive enzymes** (see page 267) with your main meal of the day. Adding pancreatic enzymes to your daily food intake not only helps temporarily to rest the digestion by taking the load off your own pancreatic function, but it can also help to control bacterial overgrowth.

- **Take supplements** that contain berberine, found in plants such as barberry bark, goldenseal and Oregon grape. In addition to being naturally antibiotic against yeasts and some bacteria, berberine inhibits the bacterial enzymes that convert proteins into the damaging vasoactive amines that I mentioned earlier. Berberine also enhances the function of immune system cells.

The importance of probiotics

When we think of bacteria, we're usually inclined to think 'yuck', bad stuff. It's true that if too many bad bugs take hold of the body, this can be the starting point for disease. But bacteria aren't all ominous. Why probiotics are helpful for so many gut disorders is still not fully understood, but research does show us that beneficial bugs have a key role to play in maintaining human health and are absolutely essential for a healthy gut. On the other hand, bacterial imbalance can mean a greater risk of disease, infection and digestive disruption. Unfortunately, most of us don't have the right bacterial balance. That's why replenishing our good bacteria is so important to our health.

Without the friendly bugs, our systems would be swamped with viral and bacterial toxins, cellular debris, chemicals, pus and bile. Beneficial bacteria transform lots of potentially nasty substances into harmless wastes ready for discharge from the body. Bile salts – an important player in the process of detoxification – are dissolved into less caustic compounds before they leave the small intestine so they don't damage the lining of the large intestine. If the good bugs are in short supply, bile can corrode the unprotected lining of the large intestine which, some observers have suggested, might cause more serious bowel disease.

Probiotics also have a hand in breaking down hormones. Again, if these good bugs are depleted, and in particular where there is a leaky gut (see page 222), primary oestrogens could be reabsorbed into the bloodstream and set up home in sensitive tissue such as that of the breast, ovary, uterus or prostate. A high level of beneficial bacteria may therefore provide us with some protection against certain types of cancer as well as against fibroids.

Jargon buster

Lactobacillus acidophilus, the long Latin name that you see on packs of yoghurt, is a natural inhabitant of the gut and, along with another probiotic, *Bifidobacterium longum*, is a major constituent in many probiotic supplements and powders. These friendly bacteria help to destroy or control harmful bacteria.

What else do probiotics do?

There is strong evidence that probiotics:

- Improve the digestion of lactose (milk sugar).
- Stimulate the immune system.
- Reduce the risk of infective diarrhoea in infants and adults.
- Reduce antibiotic-induced diarrhoea.
- Reduce the proliferation of undesirable bacteria. Most importantly, they help to prevent colonisation of the gut by those unfriendly bacteria.
- Control and limit the growth of intestinal yeasts and parasites.
- Reduce the recurrence rate of vaginal infections and decrease discharge.
- Feed on dietary fibre to create substances that can then be used for energy production by the gut.
- Help regulate the contracting and relaxing of the gut wall (peristalsis).

- Improve the consistency of faeces.

- Reduce the unpleasant odour of faeces.

- Reduce the symptoms of food allergy/intolerance.

- Manufacture some B vitamins and folic acid.

They may also be able to:

- Lower LDL cholesterol.

- Help protect us against some types of cancer.

- Improve the absorption of minerals.

Probiotic, antibiotic: what's the difference?

Well, first of all, think about the word antibiotic. It translates as 'against life'. So probiotic, it's easy to work out, means 'for life'. Probiotic bacteria are natural inhabitants of our intestines. As we've seen above, they have quite a few important jobs to do, all of which are designed to keep us healthy. If probiotic levels are consistently high, the chance of an infection taking hold is much reduced. Even if we pick up a bug of some kind, our immune system can handle it so well that we probably don't notice any symptoms.

When the levels of probiotics are reduced or damaged, the body's resistance is much lower. If an opportunist bug finds its way in, we're not so capable of fighting it off and are more likely to need a medical prescription of antibiotics to destroy the invading bacteria. There's nothing wrong with that if we really need these drugs in an emergency. Unfortunately, however, most types of antibiotic cannot distinguish between the dangerous bacteria that they are supposed to be wiping out and the friendly flora that we'd rather hang on to. So they fire indiscriminately at everything. Any amount of probiotic that we might still have had in our intestines is obliterated along with the infection.

Another result of this 'wipe out' is that the yeast *Candida albicans* (see page 65), which is normally present in every gut in small amounts, grabs the opportunity to multiply and, if left unchecked, change its structure to a more invasive type of organism. This is another reason why maintaining consistently high levels of friendly flora is such an important part of maintaining human health.

Probiotics are not new

Nor is the research behind them. The discovery that certain types of bacteria could contribute to the health of the intestines and help to ward off disease was first made way back in 1908 by a Russian scientist, Eli Metchnikoff. He was the first to use the term *dysbiosis*, to indicate an imbalance of gut bacteria. We use the word *symbiosis* to indicate that intestinal bugs are living in harmony. Since then, more than a thousand papers have been published demonstrating the benefits of friendly flora. In fact, so safe and so helpful are probiotics that, in a number of countries, doctors routinely prescribe them to repopulate the gut after antibiotics.

In the United Kingdom (surprise, surprise), this is not common practice, even though there is considerable evidence that the presence of probiotics in the gut exerts health benefits way beyond those of ordinary nutrition. Of particular interest with regard to antibiotics are studies showing that the intestines of people who receive probiotics such as *Lactobacillus acidophilus* and *Bifidobacterium bifidum* (also referred to as *B. longum and B. lactis*) recolonise more quickly than the intestines of those who do not. Happily, probiotics are available without prescription.

What causes depletion of probiotics?

Ageing, consistently poor diet, ongoing negative stress, environmental pollution and some medicines, especially antibiotics, are just a few of the things that can reduce the levels of beneficial bugs. Opportunistic infections, overgrowth of yeast organisms and attacks of infective or travellers' diarrhoea can also upset the balance. So, too, can any change of internal environment caused by inflammation, the use of spermicides, diseases of the gut and surgery.

Who needs probiotics?

I should think there are very few people who wouldn't benefit from taking regular courses of probiotics. Certainly, anyone who suffers from a chronic digestive complaint or bowel disorder of the kind that is described in this book would do themselves no harm by investing in a three-month course of top-quality probiotics, say, every twelve months. I would suggest that you take them if:

- You've just finished taking antibiotics.

- You're waiting for a doctor's appointment and think that they may prescribe antibiotics. Take probiotics beforehand but stop as soon as you begin the antibiotics and then restart them after the antibiotics course is completed. Although some experts recommend continuing probiotics alongside antibiotics, my view has always been that your antibiotics are more than likely to destroy the friendly flora along with the bacteria they are designed to kill which, let's face it, is expensive and wasteful. That's why I suggest recommencing the probiotics on the day you complete your antibiotics course and continuing for three months.

- You have a sensitive stomach and are prone to travellers diarrhoea.

- You have candidiasis or thrush or vaginal infections.

- You have repeated attacks of cystitis.

- You suffer regularly from infections.

- You have 'athlete's foot' or fungal infections of the nails or in the mouth.

- You suffer from lactose intolerance.

- You have irritable bowel syndrome.

- You suffer from food allergies.

- You're under unrelenting stress.

- You eat meat or dairy products regularly.

- You suffer regularly from dyspepsia or bloating.

- You're constipated.

- You are waiting for or recovering from an operation.

Why not just eat yoghurt?

Although some yoghurts have extra *Lactobacillus acidophilus* and other friendly bacteria added, the yoghurt itself is pasteurised which may render it less effective than concentrated probiotic supplements. However, eating yoghurt that contains live culture is an excellent dietary move, especially if you have any of the conditions detailed above.

The terrain is everything

Although it can be important to take a regular course of probiotics, swallowing supplements isn't the only move you need to make. One of the best ways of keeping probiotics happy is to create the best possible environment in the intestines.

*Pre*biotic foods are those that help to feed *Lactobacillus* bacteria and their friends. I guess you could call them a kind of Greenpeace for the gut. Some of the best dietary sources include:

- Asparagus
- Globe and Jerusalem artichokes
- All the allium family including onions, leeks, shallots, garlic and chives
- Bananas
- Endive (chicory)
- Foods rich in polyphenols (see page 100), such as ginseng and green tea, are known to have a beneficial effect on intestinal flora, increasing the good bugs and decreasing the bad ones.
- Fermented/cultured foods such as:
    - Sheep's or goat's milk yoghurt
    - Organic cottage cheese
    - Buttermilk
    - Kefir
    - Sauerkraut
    - Tempeh, miso and tamari, all made from fermented soya beans
    - Kimchee, pickled cabbage
    - Pickled daikon radish
    - Fermented milk drinks such as those made by Yakult and Danone
    - Molkosan

Some notes on Molkosan

Add a little Molkosan to fruit juices and salad dressings, and take a teaspoon in a glass of water at mealtimes. This naturally fermented lactic acid whey has a positive effect on intestinal flora, contributing not only to the reduction of unfriendly bacteria, but also to the establishment of an environment supportive to the growth of friendly bacteria. It's not enough to weed out the bad guys: you must also feed the good guys or they won't survive. Molkosan was created by Alfred Vogel, who studied extensively the history of Swiss whey cures. Whey contains all the mineral nutrients of milk without the fat and protein, and has an excellent record in the cure of intestinal complaints, flatulence and disturbed intestinal bacteria.

VERY IMPORTANT POINT

Although whey products are not usually recommended for people with lactose intolerance, in the case of Molkosan the lactose has been digested in the fermentation process and does not appear to cause any such problems. However, for the avoidance of doubt, if you are a sufferer take a tiny amount first to test for tolerance. Molkosan should never be taken neat; always dilute it.

Help to discourage bad bacteria by:

- Doing what you can to steer clear of added sugar and sugary foods. Sugar simply creates adverse conditions that encourage overgrowth of yeasts, which then put yet more strain on the levels of friendly flora that have to try and deal with it.

- Avoiding foods that contain or are made with yeast, for the same reason.

- Avoiding non-organic sources of poultry, eggs and meat. They may contain traces of the antibiotics and other drugs that are administered or added to animal feed. There is supposed to be a 'waiting time' between drug administration and slaughter, but it's strongly believed that drug residues still find their way into the food chain. Any amount of antibiotic, however small, is a potential risk to the healthy bacteria in the gut.

- Managing without cow's milk. Unless it's organic, milk too can contain traces of antibiotics that may further disrupt friendly flora. In addition, the high lactose content of milk encourages the overgrowth of *Candida albicans*, which then puts yet more strain on a healthy gut.

VERY IMPORTANT POINTS

1. **Buy the best-quality probiotics** you can afford. More often than not, products that seem like real bargains don't have the quality or the level of bacteria in them to make a difference. As a very general rule, more expensive brands are likely to have a greater level of research and development behind them, having been more extensively tested and studied than cheaper brands, and subjected to clinical trials on humans. The result is more stable strains of probiotic bacteria that are able to survive their journey through the stomach juices, which means more beneficial organisms get to where they are needed (in the small and, especially, the large intestine). Look out for quality labels such as Solgar, Viridian, Biocare, Blackmores, Higher Nature, Udo's Choice, Kiki-Health and Pharma Nord. The Resource Directory (see page 323) has stockist information.

2. **Going away?** If you're susceptible to tummy trouble, or your bowel has a tendency to tantrums, and you're going overseas to areas where there may be a higher risk of travellers' diarrhoea, I would suggest taking a course of probiotics before you leave and packing enough for while you're away. There's a lot of information available that suggests that travellers who take probiotics are less likely to be affected by food-borne bugs, diarrhoea and constipation than those that don't.

3. **Look after them** If you're taking your probiotics supplement to warmer climes, check the label for a brand that is designed to survive at ambient temperatures. Solgar, Ecozone and Higher Nature all sell probiotics that don't require refrigeration. However, this doesn't mean that they will work if subjected to extremes of heat or exposure to oxygen, so keep your supplements away from direct sunlight and replace the cap on the bottle securely after each use.

4. **When to take your probiotics** Twenty to thirty minutes before meals is best, unless the label tells you specifically to do otherwise. One of the big hurdles for most probiotics is surviving the acidic conditions of the stomach and not being destroyed before they reach their destination in the intestines. Some brands are designed to be taken with food.

26.

Essential Extras:
Digestion and Stress

He sows hurry and reaps indigestion.
Robert Louis Stevenson, *c.* 1876

Stress means different things to different people. Stress can be exciting and enjoyable (a holiday, a wedding, watching or taking part in an exhilarating sports event) or just plain bad news (rushing and *still* missing the train, being held up in traffic, falling ill or losing your credit cards). When we're suffering from stress, we tend to think in terms of how it affects us mentally or emotionally, but prolonged and unrelenting negative stress can cause just as many physical health problems as can poor diet and lack of exercise put together.

When we eat in a mad rush, or when we're anxious or angry, digestion is severely disturbed. That's because the system perceives any stressful situation as a potential crisis and clicks to 'emergency mode'. The body switches over to the section of the nervous system responsible for self-preservation – those 'fright, fight and flight' responses – and switches off the connections that are in charge of moving food through the gut and of secreting digestive enzymes. Your stomach shuts down. Blood that would normally be pumping around your digestive organs is redirected to your brain, heart and muscles, ready to fire you with quick-thinking energy in case you need to run or face the enemy. Hormones are released that thicken your blood, a safety mechanism to reduce the risk of bleeding to death if you're injured – by the dinosaur or the tiger. Your head brain moves into top gear so that decision making is sharp and speedy. Your bowel brain turns off.

Unfortunately, although you may not always be aware of it, exactly the same panic alarm is triggered in response to modern-day stressors, such as an argument, a near-squeak in the car, being late for an appointment or psyching yourself up for a visit to the dentist, as the one that is switched on in response to life-threatening situations. Noisy neighbours, money worries, concerns about your health, all these are seen as stressful events by the body, too.

The alarm phase may be short-lived, but that isn't the end of the stress. The body then moves into what's known as the resistance reaction, which allows you to carry on fighting (or running) long after the initial trigger has worn off. At this point, you'll be churning out additional adrenal hormones to help you convert proteins into energy, and to keep your blood glucose and your blood pressure high. The immune system stays fully charged in case you pick up an infection or are injured, and the brain pours chemicals into the bloodstream to help you cope with the emotional upheaval caused by the danger you are facing.

This is all well and good in a genuine emergency, but unrelenting stress and permanently extended resistance reactions are, at best – if you can call it that – an inevitable precursor to complete exhaustion and, at worst, damaging to your long-term health, leaving you at greater risk of serious disease. You have to ask yourself if the stress you are putting yourself under is really worth all this.

In addition to the damaging effects that stress has on all parts of the body, the chances are fairly high that your digestion will be affected – even if you don't notice any particular symptoms. If you're already suffering from some kind of digestive or bowel disorder, then the effects of ongoing stress can be even more damaging. Nowhere is this more obvious than in the stress-related symptoms of irritable bowel syndrome, or the acidity associated with ulcers or reflux disease. It may also be a factor in leaky gut syndrome. Stress, it seems, reduces levels of antibodies known as secretory IgA, which help to protect the gut wall from invaders (see also page 296). With this protection system compromised, the mucous membranes become more permeable and more inflamed, and the body more susceptible to attack by bacteria, yeasts and other unwanted substances, all bent on aggravating your immunity and worsening your food allergies.

Remember that I said that your gut is the first area to lose its blood supply when you're under stress? Well, did you know that the lining of your intestines is being repaired and replaced on a constant basis? If you're under permanent and unrelenting stress, the blood supply to that area can be starved, disturbing the normal process of repair.

Now I know what you're going to say. 'I'm the proverbial runaway train. I have too many commitments; they're all unavoidable and time-consuming. Too many other people rely on me. Most of the time, I get to bedtime and realise that I've done nothing for myself all day. So please don't tell me to give myself some personal space, to stand and stare or let up and let go. I don't have . . . well, I don't have the time.'

No, well, actually, I don't either so I'm not going to preach. I probably understand you better than you think. I hope you've noticed throughout this book that I've never admonished or criticised, never said you *must* do this or that. There's no point and, anyhow, I've been there myself. You're talking to the world champion workaholic here. I really do understand what it's like trying to do two or three full-time jobs, care for others and keep the home running all at the same time. If it's any consolation, I've not been a good example of how to live a stressless life. But then who is?

What I *have* discovered with age and experience is that life doesn't actually run any more smoothly if you never stop running to keep up. In fact, it's the opposite. Slowing down, breathing more deeply and count-ing to ten doesn't waste time or delay you; it restores your perspective and calms you so that your judgement improves and your precious time is better spent. Truly. The problem we all have is making the change from barmy to balmy. More often than not, that change is nothing more than one of attitude. So, for a change, practise some stress-busting instead of stress-building.

Look at it this way. When you're not here anymore, will it have mattered if you rushed to that appointment, got steamed up about the parking ticket, skipped lunch, flew around the supermarket, grabbed a bar of chocolate on the way home, ate your supper standing up in the kitchen, spent the evening working and fell asleep before your head hit the pillow? Well? Will it? Will any of it matter in a hundred years' time?

No, of course it won't. Stress is not, I'm sure you've realised by now, caused by any particular event or experience but by how you perceive that situation. Change your perception and some things – not all, of course – but quite a few things that you used to see as terribly stressful can become just ordinary occurrences. A quick for instance?

You're following a car that is slow and hesitating. You make several attempts to overtake it (one of the most stressful driving manoeuvres, by the way) and eventually manage to get past, only to get caught behind a farm vehicle chugging along at 40 kilometres (25 miles) an hour. The road is twisty and you can't see ahead. You can feel your palms getting sticky and your breathing becoming erratic. There's an odd kind of pressure in your chest. By the time you get to where you're going, you feel awful. You may have heartburn or stomach ache, or urgent diarrhoea. You need to stop, to 'settle' your nerves, except you haven't got the time.

So what was it all for? Did you save anything by playing 'kissing bumpers' with the vehicle in front. Would it have made any difference to your day if you'd just accepted the delay, put on a CD or the radio in the car, left some space, taken in the scenery and enjoyed the trip? Remember the old Zen saying that the early bird may get the worm, but the second mouse gets the cheese in the trap.

I stopped worrying about traffic delays the day I was held up by one of those wide loads on a really busy road where there was no opportunity to overtake. I followed it for mile upon mile until everything came to a stop because, up ahead, there was a nasty road accident. There were four police cars, two fire engines and three ambulances. I had this really strong gut feeling that if I'd managed to get by the wide load earlier, I'd almost certainly have been driving faster and could well have been involved in the accident too. To me it was a message, a warning, if you like, to slow down, not just in my car but in my life, too. So I did. Now I poodle along and get there just the same. Boring? Maybe. But safer and healthier as a result.

These are just a few of the physical symptoms that can be associated with unrelenting pressure. How many of them apply to you?

Acid reflux	Muscle spasms
Body odour	Nail biting
Chronic fatigue	Neck tension
Attacks of diarrhoea	Overactive mind
Food cravings	Palpitations
Headaches	Poor coordination
High blood pressure	Reduced resistance to infections
Indigestion or heartburn	Restless limbs
Insomnia	Sour breath
Jaw pain	Stomach cramps
Joint pain	Sweating
Lack of – or increased – appetite	Tearfulness
Loss of libido	Teeth grinding
Migraine	Tight shoulders
More colds	

I hope that reading through this list might make you want to make the change. Adopt a 'positive thinking' approach like that recommended by Louise Hay in her famous book *You Can Heal Your Life*. Don't be depressed by the weather, she says. It's not a foul day, it's just a wet day. There is, we know but all tend to forget, sunshine behind every cloud.

We also forget how important it is to relax. We might try for a day or two and then, when life gets in the way, give up. Yet managing stress and learning how to relax are both important factors in maintaining a healthy digestion. They can seem hard to achieve at the outset but practice really does make perfect. No one is suggesting or expecting that you'll suddenly become a faultless and stress-free manager. It can't be done and it wouldn't be natural. Some stress is good for us. But don't allow yourself to be overwhelmed by *overstress*. This can happen when sadness engulfs happiness, a negative state that could actually physically damage your digestion.

Balance is the key

Do what you can to introduce one or two changes each week and stick to them. And then congratulate yourself on your progress.

Before you begin . . .

Think hard about what worries you. If you're suffering from any kind of stomach or digestive disorder, it might be helpful to consider the following:

- Do you feel aggressive or angry towards someone or something? If the answer is yes, try to analyse why this might be.

- Is something 'eating away at you'?

- Is there something that you're finding hard to swallow?

- Are you good, or not so good, at handling your feelings?

- Are you ignoring your *gut* feelings?

- Is there something you're afraid of?

- Is it a known fear or a fear of the unknown?

- Is there a new experience that you're finding it hard to assimilate?

- Are you happy with (can you stomach) who you are?

- Are you fed up with being the strong one, the one who copes?

- Do you wish you could go back to your childhood or to somewhere without conflict or pressure?

- Do you ever have that weird feeling that you're lost in familiar territory, or you're viewing your world from the sidelines? The unpleasant sensation of being 'spaced out' – so often associated with persistent negative stress – can be difficult to put into words but was once described to me as being diagonally parked in a parallel universe.

This simple self-analysis can often put problems and stressful events into perspective. If you've suffered severe emotional trauma that could be affecting your health, then could you benefit from seeing a clinical psychologist or psychotherapist? Talk to your doctor about a referral. And don't be afraid to ask; the service is there to help you. Rest assured that you're not alone and you're not the only one who feels this way. You're certainly not 'going mad' or 'losing it'. Everyone is affected by fear and trepidation; it's simply that some of us are more susceptible than others. If a problem seems insurmountable, ask for help. It isn't a crime or a weakness to need other people. If your doctor is unsympathetic, don't take it personally. Change doctors or ask for a referral.

Take care of *you*

If you're exposed to excessive stress, you need to take extra special care of yourself. Living with stress is not good for your physical or emotional health. That digestive or bowel problem could be a signal for help. Do something about it before it overwhelms you and you develop something more serious than an irritable colon or acid stomach.

Laugh yourself better

The first thing you need to do is treat yourself to a change of mood. Ever noticed how it's always harder to cope if your perspective is out of kilter, usually when you're feeling miserable, hard done by, bored or exhausted? Begin by introducing things into your life that make you laugh. If you hire or buy a DVD or a video, go for humour, not horror. Watch good comedy on television. Read works by writers who have a sense of humour, such as Maureen Lipman, Bill Bryson, Ivor Cutler, Des McHale or Rohan Candappa. Be with friends who know how to have fun. Steer clear of bores who flatten your mood. Not only can laughing make you feel better, instantly, but it can also be a cure, all by itself. Even the simple act of smiling, to other people or to yourself, can send positive messages to your cells. If you find this hard to believe, try smiling now and see how it makes you feel. Laughter improves your circulation and your intake of oxygen, lifts depression and helps you cope more easily with the negative aspects of daily living. Laughing is also a way of 'letting go', something that can be of particular benefit to people who suffer from constipation.

Beware
Don't rely on stimulants to conceal your stress
Resorting to coffee, cola drinks, sugary and sweet foods, alcohol and ciga-rettes are the negative moves that some people make to cope with stress. They're quick lift options if you're flagging, hungry or need consolation. Bombing out in front of the TV, comfort eating, overspending on shopping or turning to drugs for support are also negative coping patterns associated with excessive stress. But there are no plus points here. You might disguise your *dis*-stress for a while but all these things actually pile on the pressure by overstimulating all body systems, *including the digestion*.

Have fun reading
Fancy a relaxing read? Not everyone appreciates the same kind of humour so it's important to choose what makes you laugh. How about *The Little Book of Bollocks* by Alistair Beaton, *The Little Book of Crap Advice* by Michael Powell, *Why Men Don't Listen & Women Can't Read Maps* by Allan and Barbara Pease or *The Ladies Room Revisited*, a compendium of amusing and interesting female facts. Indulge yourself in *It's A Long Way From Penny Apples* by Bill Cullen or *Billy* by Pamela Stephenson. Or immerse yourself in some classic comedy such as *The Complete Yes Minister* by Jonathan Lynn and Anthony Jay, or perhaps the works of Stephen Fry or Ben Elton. Or, one of my particular favourites, *Down Under* by Bill Bryson (although Australians may not agree).

Realise that you are important

The second fundamental is to learn to give yourself priority. This isn't *selfish*, this is *self-care*. Stop multi-tasking. Don't get into that guilt trip that says you don't have the time. Be polite, be firm and say 'no' every now and then.

Treat yourself

Appreciate the importance of treating yourself. Whether it's a home manicure, a weekly or monthly visit to the beauty salon or the hair-dresser, make time for pampering you. Invest in a regular session of re-flexology, an aromatherapy massage, an Indian head massage or shiatsu. If you're a coiled spring, consider learning how to meditate, or taking classes in yoga, t'ai chi, or chi gong. Don't think of these as occasional treatments or as luxuries but as health insurance – relaxing *and* thera-peutic. And don't forget that self-massage of the scalp, neck, hands, feet and abdomen are all destressing and relaxing.

Count your blessings

Remember how lucky you are. Counting your blessings may be an old-fashioned remedy for stress and anxiety but it's one that works. Life can seem dismal and desperate when you're struggling with a difficult job, or when everything seems to be going wrong or if there isn't enough money for what you want. But if you have shoes on your feet, clothes on your back, a roof over your head and enough to eat, then everything else is surely a bonus? If you have family or friends who would be sad if you weren't around, you have great riches.

Take time out

Diarise your leisure time just as you do your appointments. And take that time off no matter what. You deserve it. We all need 'wind-down' time to gather our thoughts, process the day's events, and let our body and mind get back into sync with each other.

Don't be a slouch

Check your posture. It's easy to get cramped and tight behind the wheel, behind the desk or in front of the VDU. A crouched, slumped position not only affects your breathing but also stresses and tenses your gut.

Respect your digestive system

Don't put it under unnecessary strain by abusing it. If you haven't already done so, read the chapter If You Do Nothing Else . . . that begins on page 250, and include as many of the tips as suit you. This section is as important to stress reduction as learning how to breathe properly. By improving the way your body digests and absorbs its food, you also up your intake of the vitamins, minerals and essential fatty acids that you need to nurture your nervous system. And it's your nervous system, you'll remember from page 199, that controls pretty much everything that goes on in your gut.

Listen to the music

Use soothing music to calm you when you're stressed, and zingy rhythmic beats to inject lost energy and get your body and mind moving along. Music also changes mood and lifts boredom, both of which can make you feel stressed.

Get moving

Daily physical activity such as walking, swimming, cycling, dancing, rebounding and skipping really does make a difference. Play golf – or just walk the course with someone else. Choose what appeals most to you. The trick is to make exercise enjoyable. Simple stretching exercises done before and after vigorous activity tone the muscles and reduce the risk of spasm and cramp.

I met someone quite recently who admitted that the only time her bowels functioned properly was during her annual walking holiday – when she was exercising every day and feeling more relaxed. Research shows that regular exercise coupled to a healthy diet containing sufficient dietary fibre can lower the risk of some bowel disorders by as much as 40 per cent. Go gently and don't do too much. Start off with fifteen to twenty minutes every day and work up to thirty minutes per day.

Learn to relax

Easier said than done? Consider yoga, or learn transcendental meditation (TM), chi gong, autogenic training or t'ai chi. It really is worth going to local classes. Ask at your adult education centre, health food store or library for information.

Do breathing exercises

Exercise your insides with regular deep-breathing exercises. Five minutes on waking and another five before settling down to sleep are usually enough to make the difference. Chinese philosophy has it that distress, anxiety and sadness lead to dysfunction of the large intestine by injuring the lungs. Improving the quality of the breathing can increase energy flow between those organs. I've seen significant improvements in patients who have introduced simple daily deep breathing exercises into their routine. Begin right now: take a deep breath and let out a big sigh. And then do it again. It's *the* remedy for releasing tension. (I'll be looking at the subject of deep breathing in more depth below, where I've also included some deep-breathing exercises.)

Eat light and nourishing food

Don't scoff down a big meal if you're very stressed or overly anxious. Soups, juices and yoghurt are gentle on a stressed digestion. Don't go for a large meal if you're rushed. Remember that stressful conditions cause the stomach to 'shut down'. Undigested or partially digested food will eventually pass through to the small intestine, causing irritation and increasing the risk of further digestive troubles.

Choose the right snacks

If you feel hungry between meals, go for easy-to-digest foods such as yog-hurt, soup, a chopped salad or some vegetable juice. Don't put up with hunger pangs just because it isn't a regulation mealtime. A light snack will boost your blood sugar and lift your energy. Missing a meal when you are already struggling with an empty stomach not only aggravates digestive discomfort, but also addles your brain and disturbs your concentration.

Give your body the support it needs

If you try to survive on snatched snacks, takeaways or packeted processed foods, your system won't have the goodness to help protect you against the ravages of negative stress. Eating the kind of balanced diet I've talked about throughout this book, concentrating on natural, unadulterated whole-foods, lean protein, beans, seeds, vegetables, dried and fresh fruits and cold-pressed oils, will provide you with essential anti-stress sustenance.

Learn to breathe more deeply

Efficient breathing is, without doubt, one of the best ways to reduce stress. Most people who are under stress have shallow, rapid breathing interspersed with sighs. If you could do with more breathing space, practise the following exercises. If you need more help, get hold of a copy of the cassette tape *Healthy Breathing* by Ken Cohen. It will provide you with a very inexpensive way to learn to breathe properly.

Before you try to change your breathing, practise moving your abdomen and diaphragm. Chest breathing, which most of us do most of the time, is really only supposed to be an emergency measure when you're under stress and need to pump air quickly in and out of the body. Diaphragmatic breathing, sometimes also referred to as abdominal breathing, is much deeper and slower. To breathe properly, you need to train yourself to take air in the lower sections of the lungs.

Diaphragmatic breathing technique

Lie down with one hand on your belly and the other on your chest. Breathe as you would normally without changing anything or trying to introduce any new techniques. I would bet that most people find that the hand on their chest rises and falls as they breathe but that the hand on the belly moves only a little or not at all. What you want to achieve is the reverse of this and one of the easiest ways of doing so is to imagine that there's a balloon inside your abdomen that fills each time you breathe in and collapses each time you breathe out. Don't worry about the *quality* of the breath at this stage. As you breathe in, push your abdomen out and up. As you breathe out, pull the abdominal muscles in so that you have curved a hollow into your lower back and under your ribcage. It will feel strange at first, but after some practice you should find that this movement will happen naturally with the consequence that you'll be breathing more deeply than before.

Breathing exercises

1. Here is a quick-to-do breathing exercise for when you first wake in the morning and for last thing at night while you're waiting to go to sleep.

- Breathe in through the nose, then let go with a big sigh.

- Breathe in through the nose, slowly and gently, allowing your abdomen to extend as far as is comfortable.

- Hold for a count of one.

- Breathe out, slowly again through the nose, as you do so trying to picture your whole body letting go.

- Repeat for ten in-breaths and ten out-breaths.

- Deep breathing helps to lower your blood pressure and increases oxygen flow throughout the body. Deep abdominal breathing should also exercise and tone your digestive system.

2. Read this next exercise straight through once and then read it again, step by step. Practise the steps three or four times, then introduce them into your daily routine whenever you feel anxious, uncomfortable, angry or tired. This is a great set that you can do at any time: at your desk, in the car, at the dining table, in the bathroom. All movements should be done very slowly, in time with the breath. Be gentle. You will achieve nothing by pushing or straining. Just move as far as you can with comfort. If it's easier for you, breathe in and out between each change of movement.

- First, take a deep breath in through the nose and exhale with a big sigh through the mouth.

- Breathe in, and as you do so, tighten and screw up the muscles in your face, pulling faces, yawning, moving the mouth from side to side and rolling the eyes.

- Then relax the face and breathe out, again through the nose. If you're in a public place and prefer not to look as though you've completely lost it, do this first part of the exercise by breathing in and out and simply trying to relax all the muscles in the face and neck without screwing them up first.

- Breathe in again and as you breathe out, relax and drop the shoulders. Continuing to breathe steadily, rotate the shoulders making circles forwards and backwards. Go very gently. Don't strain.

- Breathe in. This time, as you exhale, move the head gently to the left so that your left ear tries to meet the top of your left shoulder. No strain is needed. Don't push too far, just move until the muscles resist and then, as you breathe in again, bring the head back up to normal position.

- Breathe out and move the head so that the right ear moves towards the right shoulder.

- Breathe in and stretch your arms out in front of you, wiggle your fingers, make circles with your hands, then clench your fists and tense your arm muscles.

- Breathe out and relax.

3. If you're lucky enough to live among that rare commodity, fresh air, this exercise is worth the practice. Stand near an open door or window with your hands behind your head and your elbows pointing forwards. As you breathe in, move the elbows to either side, opening out the chest. Stretch gently and hold for one second. When breathing out, move your elbows so that they are pointing forwards again. Pace the elbow movements with the breath. This can be a particular helpful exercise for those who spend a lot of time behind the wheel or work in front of VDU screens. Driving and keyboard work both encourage a slouched posture, cramping the chest and encouraging indigestion.

4. Practising what is known as progressive relaxation is one of the best ways of making a stressed body aware of how tense it actually is. Apart from being an effective way of helping the body to relax, it also helps to relieve anxiety, release anger and improve quality of sleep. This exercise is best done in the prone position on a comfortable mat on the floor, stretched fully out on a sofa or on a bed. Before you begin, loosen any tight clothing, and make sure you are comfortable and not likely to be disturbed. Support your head and neck with a cushion or pillow or rolled up towel. It can also help to cover the eyes. A wash-cloth or large cotton handkerchief, soaked in cool water and squeezed out, blocks out the light, helps concentration and, as a bonus, rests the eyes and reduces puffiness.

- First of all, do the ten in-breaths and ten out-breaths suggested in Exercise 1.

- Breathe in and out through the nose.

- Next, take a deep breath in and exhale with a big sigh.

- As you breathe in again, curl and tighten your toes, raising your feet up towards your ankles.

- Hold for a count of three, breathe out and let go.

- Breathe in again and, this time, tense the muscles in your calves, backs of knees and thighs.

- Hold for a count of three, breathe out and let go.

- Now pay attention to your buttocks, hips, pelvic area and abdomen, tightening all the muscles in these parts of the body as you breathe in.

- Hold for a count of three, breathe out and let go.

- Now think about your back. Tense your upper torso and chest area as you breathe in.

- Hold for a count of three, breathe out and let go.

- Now move to your shoulders, breathing in and squeezing your arms into your body.

- Hold for a count of three, breathe out and let go.

- Next time you breathe in, tighten your neck muscles and all the muscles in your face (the easiest way to do this is to imagine you can smell an unpleasant smell that is making you screw up your nose and forehead).

- Hold for a count of three, breathe out and let go.

- Finally, breathe in really slowly and brace your whole body so that you are tense from the tips of your toes to the top of your head.

- Hold for a count of three, breathe out and let go.

Be aware of how relaxed you feel. Stay with the steady breathing and repeat these words to yourself (out loud if possible), three times:

'I am **relaxed**; I am **comfortable**; I am **safe**.'

Breathe in again and introduce one of the following lines with each out-breath:

1. 'I release and let go of all **tension**.'
2. 'I release and let go of all **anger**.'
3. 'I release and let go of all **guilt**.'
4. 'I release and let go of all **resentment**.'

5. 'I release and let go of all **fear**.'
6. 'I release and let go of all **pain and discomfort**.'

Picture all those negative emotions discharging from your body and then repeat:

'I am **relaxed**; I am **comfortable**; I am **safe**.'

Be aware of how much calmer you feel now than when you first began this exercise.

Regular relaxation leads not only to reduced stress and less tension but also to a calmer mind. Let your mind drift and imagine your body floating. This level of relaxation takes practice and doesn't always come easily first time. It's taken me a good long time to learn how to achieve deep relaxation on cue, but that's what happens if you keep on practising. Then, when you do get stressed or anxious or don't feel so well, you've already trained your body to recognise that deep breathing is the signal to slow down, clear the clutter from your overly active brain and immerse yourself in peaceful, safe and private surroundings.

Tips to get you through a stressful day

Eat breakfast

Sorry to sound like everyone's grandmother, but it really is the most important meal of the day. Skipping breakfast results in your blood glucose levels being low at the start of the day, your low attention span, poor concentration (more risk of having an accident on the way to work or school) and your adrenal glands, which are already overworked, simply getting overworked some more.

Munch a healthy lunch

Skipping lunch may seem like a time saver but all it does is short change your health.

Let fluid out and take fluid in

Empty your bladder, rinse your hands and face, then get yourself a drink of herbal or green tea, fresh juice or plain water. Chamomile tea is calming and good for the digestion.

Give your feet a rest

Take off your shoes, wiggle your toes and rub your feet and ankles. If your feet ache, your shoes pinch or your legs are tired, you could be putting extra strain on your whole system. In reflexology, points on the feet relate to the organs of the body. Firm massage over the whole of the foot, in particular the arch and the heel, will cover most of the points that relate to the digestive system. Rubbing the reflex points yourself is unlikely to have the long-term benefits of an experienced and talented reflexologist but can certainly provide short-term relief.

Switch off your phone

Always wired to your mobile? Switch it off and be unavailable once in a while. The world won't end.

Use a face spray

Give yourself an instant lift with a face spray. Keep a pocket-sized spray in your handbag or next to your computer. Terrific if you're stressed, tired, bored or hot, or if your brain needs a burst of energy. Use a water-only mister such as Evian or choose one that contains essential oils. Jurlique Clarity Blend is good if your perspective needs rejigging. Go for Jurlique Tranquility Blend if you're anxious or need calming. Not pocket-sized but inexpensive and refreshing is Lifestream Biogenic Aloe Vera Mist from Xynergy Health, a mix of aloe vera with vitamin E and witch hazel. These are just a few of my favourites. A chemist or beauty counter will have lots more to choose from.

Massage your ears

It can improve mood and lift energy. Using fingers and thumb, start at the lobes and work up to the top. This way you'll cover all the acupuncture points that relate to the rest of the body.

Get some fresh air

Open the windows or stand outside for a couple of minutes. Lose yourself in the view or, if you don't have a good one, close your eyes for a couple of minutes and visualise a favourite place.

Stretch

Follow this simple routine. Twirl your ankles: first one, clockwise and anti-clockwise, then the other, in both directions. Next, breathing in, lift your arms up from your sides and raise them above your head. Stretch so you can feel a gentle pull in your chest and abdomen. As you breathe out, return your arms to the sides. Next, think shoulders. Breathing in, lift up the shoulders – slowly and gently – towards your ears, then breathe out with a big sigh, letting the shoulders flop. Breathe in. Tip your head slowly to one side so that your left ear moves towards your left shoulder. Don't strain. As you do this, breathe out. Then breathe in, lifting your head back to the centre. Then the other way – right ear to right shoulder, breathing out. Slowly does it. Back to the centre. Straighten up and breathe in. Keeping the head level and with your eyes looking forwards (so your head moves and your eyes don't) breathe out, moving the head to the left. Breathe in and return to the centre. Breathe out and move to the right. Breathe in and return to the centre. Relax.

Wash away your stress

A luxurious soak or invigorating shower can help to wash away the stresses of the day. Be completely unavailable, lock the door, play your favourite music, and make use of calming essential oils such as lavender, frankincense or sandalwood, either in the water or via a burner or vaporiser, then treat yourself to some delicious skin-care products.

Use essential oils

A few drops of essential oil sloshed around in the bath water can be an instant destresser. Lavender and Roman chamomile are especially calming. Pine is stimulating and strengthening. Rosemary will refresh and revive and, like ginger, is a traditional remedy for digestive complaints. Clary sage is balancing. Thyme oil relieves anxiety. Frankincense restores perspective and is good if your stress is making you apprehensive or nervous. Orange and lemon essential oils are the ones to choose if you're feeling negative. Always dilute pure oils into a carrier oil before use. Buy quality oils such as Jurlique, Nelsons or Tisserand. *Aromatherapy Stress Management* by Christine Westwood is an excellent and inexpensive guide to home use of essential oils.

Take herbs to calm your nerves

If you're really struggling to cope during the day or stress is keeping you awake at night, a herbal supplement based on passion flower, oats, hops, Californian poppy or valerian can be a non-addictive alternative to tranquillisers. Ask your health food store, herbalist or pharmacist for advice. Herbal remedies are not quick fixes but, in conjunction with good nutrition, regular exercise and stress-reducing lifestyle changes, they can help you through the bad patches.

Helpful hint

If sleep eludes you, try one of these herbal remedies: Bioforce Passiflora Complex, Kiwiherb Valerian Root Extract, Nitebalm (from Natural Woman), Blackmores Passiflora Complex or Valerian or Passiflora from Arkopharma. Sedonium from Lichtwer Pharma is available from most pharmacy counters. NT188 capsules (Biocare) contains magnesium and passion-flower extract to help nourish the nervous system and encourage quality sleep. And if you're having one of those days when nothing goes right, try Arkopharma's Californian Poppy; I've found it a really useful daytime remedy for stress.

Drink herbal teas

Instead of coffee, introduce herbal teas. If, like me, you're not a fan of most herbal teas, you can still benefit from them. I've grown to like them all by adding a squeeze of fresh lemon or lime juice, a slice of fresh root ginger and half a teaspoon of Comvita Manuka honey to them. Peppermint, chamomile and ginger teas are all good for the digestion. Lemon balm and limeflower tea is an old remedy for insomnia and is an excellent calmer just before bedtime. As a special treat, try one of the Jurlique range of herbal teas. My favourites include Pick-Me-Up, After Meal Feel Good and Good Night Sweet Dreams, and the All Root Blend, which is also great for the digestion.

And finally...

Read *Stress Busters* by Robert Holden. It's still one of the best destressing books around.

VERY IMPORTANT POINT

Stress is unavoidable but it doesn't have to rule our lives. The ability to relax and to calm the mind and the body is an absolutely essential prerequisite not only for relieving the effects of existing stress but also for helping the system to cope with the stresses yet to come.

Reducing stress

KATHRYN'S TOP TEN TIPS

1. Consider the care of yourself a priority.

2. Adopt a positive attitude.

3. Eat a nourishing diet.

4. Stop for regular meals.

5. Cut back on – and find alternatives to – coffee, alcohol and sugar.

6. Take supplements to top up your diet and support your adrenal system.

7. Take exercise at least three times a week.

8. Deal with relationship issues.

9. Learn to breathe properly and practise progressive relaxation.

10. Get plenty of sleep.

www.teachhealth.com This fun site is also educational and informative. Sensible advice on how to survive stress.

www.stressbusting.com has some valuable stress-busting strategies.

www.theflow.org When the site opens up, click on Chinese Chi Kung Meditations. And then look at the each of the options to the left of the screen. Listen to the audio samples and follow the exercises. Introduce some of them into your daily routine and see if you don't feel better.

Resource Directory

Useful Addresses

Independent health food stores should stock most of the items recommended in Good Gut Healing. To find your nearest stockist or to order by post, use the contact list below.

Arkopharma, 7 Redlands Centre, Coulsdon, Surrey CR5 2HT
Telephone 020 8763 1414
Write with your name and address for price list and order form or e-mail sales@arkopharma.co.uk
More information at
www.arkopharma.com/english
Wide range of herbal supplements. Cold-pressed flax oil liquid and capsules.

Biocare, Lakeside, 180 Lifford Lane, Kings Norton, Birmingham B30 3NT
Telephone 0121 433 3727
Fax: 0121 433 3879
www.biocare.co.uk
Wide range of vitamin, mineral and herbal products. Specialists in digestive enzymes, probiotics.

Bioforce, 2 Brewster Place, Irvine, Ayrshire KA11 5DD
Telephone Helpline 0845 6085858
www.bioforce.co.uk
Herbal medicines, echinacea drops, Silicea liquid, Organic food seasonings, Papayaforce, Organic herbal tinctures and tablets, Alfred Vogel's Swiss Muesli, Jan de Vries Bowel Essence

Bio-Health, Medway City Estate, Rochester, Kent ME2 4HU
Telephone 01634 290115
Quality herbal medicines.

Blackmores UK Ltd., c/o Apotheke 20-20, 300-302 Chiswick High Rd, London W2H 1PA
Telephone 020 8995 2293
Blackmores Bio-C tablets, Milk Thistle, Digestive Aid, Colon Care, Acidophilus & Bifidus, Garlix, Executive B Formula, Echinacea Forte 3000, Slippery Elm tablets, Celloid Minerals.

Blackmores Australia, 23 Roseberry Street, Balgowlah NSW 2093
Telephone 02 9951 0111
Fax 02 9949 1954
webmaster@blackmores.com.au

Blackmores New Zealand, PSM Healthcare Ltd., 14–16 Norman Spencer Drive, Manukau City, Auckland.
Telephone 09 279 7979
Fax 09 279 7999   sales@psm.co.nz

Blackmores Singapore, Neucor Holdings Pte Ltd., No. 10 Upper Aljunied Link, # 05–12 York International Industrial Building, Singapore 367904
Telephone 65 6280 1169
Fax 65 6285 4515   lynette@neucor.com

Complementary Medicine Services, 9 Corporation Street, Taunton, Somerset TA1 4AJ
Telephone 'advice desk' 01823 325022
Telephone orders 01823 321027
Allergy Care brochure. Specialist suppliers of foods for people suffering from allergies.

Delamere Dairy, Yew Tree Farm, Bexton Lane, Knutsford, Cheshire WA16 9BH
Telephone 01565 632422
wwwdelameredairy.co.uk
info@delameredairy.co.uk
Wide range of goat's milk products including cheeses and yoghurts. Avaliable from most major supermarkets.

E-Cloth System, EnviroProducts Ltd, The Brewery, Bells Yew Green, Tunbridge Wells, Kent TN3 9BD
Telephone 01892 752199
info@enviroproducts.co.uk
www.e-cloth.com
Range of cleaning cloths and mops which work without household chemicals. Great cloths anyway, but especially good if you suffer allergies or multiple chemical sensitivities. Available by mail from the manufacturer and from Lakeland Limited 01539 488100;
www.lakelandlimited.co.uk

Also from retail outlets such as John Lewis, Waitrose, Comet, Currys, B & Q, and independent DIY and hardware stores.

Ecozone, Unit 1, Tannery Close, Beckenham, Kent BR3 4BY
Telephone 0208 662 7200
Fax 0208 662 7222   info@ecozone.co.uk
www.ecozone.co.uk
Specialist in eco-friendly products. Enzymes, probiotics.
Stockist for Green People and Biocare.

Enviroproducts Ltd., The Brewery, Bell's Yew Green, Tunbridge Wells, Kent TN3 9BD
Telephone 01892 752199
www.e-cloth.uk.com
Range of amazing cloths for all kinds of household cleaning that work without the need for chemicals.

Foods Matter **at the Inside Story**, The Inside Story, Berrydale House, 5 Lawn Road, London NW3 2XS
A quarterly newsletter containing useful articles, recipes, latest findings and an extensive list of self-help and support groups, valuable to anyone suffering from food allergies or food intolerances. Highly recommended. Write enclosing a large stamped addressed envelope for subscription details.

G&G Vitamin Shop, Vitality House, 2–3 Imberhorne Way, East Grinstead, West Sussex RH19 1RL
Telephone 01342 312811
www.gandgvitamins.com
Digestive Complex, green walnut tincture, clove capsules, Wormwood capsules.

Green People Company, Brighton Road, Handcross, West Sussex RH17 6BZ
Telephone 01444 401444
www.greenpeople.co.uk
Organic Omega 3&6 flax/pumpkin/borage oil mix, Organic Omega 3&6 flax seed sprinkle, organic skin-care products. *See also* Ecozone.

Healthy House, The Old Co-op, Ruscombe, Stroud,

Gloucestershire GL6 6BU
Telephone 01453 752216
info@healthy-house.co.uk
www.healthy-house.co.uk
E-mail, write or phone for product brochure. Specialist products for people with allergies.

Higher Nature, The Nutrition Centre, Burwash Common, East Sussex TN19 7LX
Telephone 01435 882880
www.higher-nature.co.uk
Details also available on food allergy testing. Excellent product brochure available. Flax seed and oil products, hemp seed oil, psyllium, probiotics, aloe vera drinks and topical gel. Cleansing products including Paraclens.

Homoeopathic Medicines, available from health food stores and by mail from Ainsworths Homoeopathic Pharmacy, 38 New Cavendish Street, London W1M 9FG
Telephone 0171 935 5330
Also from Neal's Yard. (See page 325).

Jurlique, NHBC Ltd., c/o Apotheke 20-20, 300-302 Chiswick High Rd, London W2H 1PA
Telephone 020 8995 2293
www.apotheke20-20.co.uk
Jurlique specialist herbal teas, organic skin-care products, essential oils.

Jurlique International, Jurlique has very extensive international distribution. Their home page is **www.jurlique.com**, and there is an international distributors page at **www.jurlique.com.au/Locations/Locations.html**.

Kiki Health, 3 Windsor Avenue, Great Yarmouth, Norfolk NR30 4EA.
Telephone 01493 857878
www.kiki-health.com
E3Live blue green algae, Nature's Biotics probiotic supplements (also available from *Natural Woman*).

Kiwiherb, Kiwiherb products are available through all independent health food stores and by mail order through Xynergy Health (see below).

www.kiwiherb.com
Meadowsweet & aniseed, ginger &
kawakawa syrup, valerian root extract,
echinacea, calendula oinment.

Kiwiherb New Zealand, 438 Rosebank
Rd, Avondale, Auckland.

Lichtwer Phama, herbal products
available from Boots, Superdrug, The Nutri
Centre and from health food stores. In case
of difficulty, telephone 01628 533307 or
visit **www.lichtwer.co.uk**

Manuka Honey Products, look for
Comvita Manuka, available from good
health food stores and by post from
Xynergy Health. In case of difficulty,
contact Xynergy or New Zealand Natural
Food Company.

Comvita New Zealand, Paengaroa, Bay
of Plenty, New Zealand.

Comvita Asia Ltd., 501 Technology
Plaza, 651 Kings Road, North Point, Hong
Kong.

Comvita USA, Pacific Resources
International, P.O. Box 668, Summerland,
CA 93067

Natural Woman Ltd., 86 Shirehampton
Road, Stoke Bishop, Bristol BS9 2DR
Telephone 0117 968 7744
www.natural-woman.com
Udo's Choice products, PelvicToner
stockist, Biocare stockist,
Nature's Biotics from Kiki Health.

**Naturopathic Health & Beauty
Company**, c/o Apotheke 20-20, 300-302
Chiswick High Rd, London W2H 1PA
Telephone 020 8995 2293
Quality skin-care products and
supplements, Jurlique products.

New Zealand Natural Food Company,
Unit 7, 55-57 Park Royal Road,
London NW10 7JP
Telephone: 0181 961 4410
www.comvita.com & www.kiwiherb.com
Products also available from Xynergy
Health.

Neal's Yard, mail order, 29 John Dalton
Street, Manchester M2 6DS
Telephone 0161 831 7875
Customer services telephone
020 7627 1949
www.nealsyardremedies.com
Homeopathic medicines. Wide range of
herbal tinctures such as echinacea and
dried herbs including slippery elm; natural
skin-care products, essential oils.

Pharma Nord, Spital Hall, Mitford,
Morpeth, Northumberland NE61 3PN
Telephone 01670 519989 or Freephone
0800 591756
Extensive range of vitamin, mineral and
other supplements, probiotics, Q10 skin-
care products.

Potters Herbal Medicines, Leyland Mill
Lane, Wigan, Lancashire WN1 2SB.
Telephone 01942 405100
www.herbal-direct.com

Raven's Oak Dairy, Burland Farm,
Wrexham Road, Burland, Nantwich,
Cheshire
Telephone 01270 524624
www.ravensoakdairy.com
info@ravensoakdairy.com
Mail order supplies of organic goat, buffalo
and sheep's milk cheeses.

St Helen's Farm,
Telephone 01430 861715
www.sthelensfarm.co.uk
Suppliers of goat's milk products including
cheeses and yoghurts. Avaliable from
Tesco, Sainsburys, Safeway and Waitrose.
Informative website with a good recipe
section.

Savant Health, Quarry House, Clayton
Wood Close, Leeds LS16 6QE
Telephone 0113 230 1993
Fax 0113 230 1915
www.savant-health.com
Udo's Choice Beyond Greens, Udo's Choice
Super 5 and Super 8 Probiotics,Udo's
Choice Digestive Enzyme Blend,Udo's
Choice Ultimate Oil Blend.

The Soil Association, Bristol House,
40–56 Victoria Street, Bristol BS1 6BY

www.soilassociation.org
Regional Guides available giving organic
producers/stockists, opening times, types
of produce sold, delivery and mail order
services county by county. Send large
stamped addressed envelope.

Solgar Vitamins, Albury, Tring,
Hertfordshire HP23 5PT
Telephone 01442 890355
www.solgar.com
Gold label range, vitamins, minerals,
enzymes, psyllium, probiotics and other
specialist supplements.

Solgar Australia, Locked Bag 5010,
Baulkham Hills, NSW 2153
Telephone 02 8858 6170
Fax 02 9023 0019
www.solgar.com.au

Solgar New Zealand, Level 1, 15 Vestey
Drive, Mount Wellington, Auckland.
Telephone 09 573 5101   Fax 09 573 0203

Solgar Singapore, Essential Living
Pte. Ltd, Blk 194 Pandan Loop,
#01–01 Pantech Indl Complex,
Singapore 128383.
Telephone: 65 6276 1380
Fax 65 6276 1370
essliv@pacific.net.sg
www.essliv.com

Solgar South Africa, P.O. Box 365,
Kya Sands, 2613 Randburg
Telephone 21 1708 3943
Fax 21 1708 1201
margalm@labs.wyeth.com

Solgar US, Solgar Vitamin and Herb,
500 Frank W. Burr Boulevard, Teaneck,
NJ 07666
Telephone 201 944 2311
Fax 201 944 7351

Spiezia Organic Care Ltd., The Barn
Workshop, Rosuick Farm, St. Martins,
Helston, Cornwall TR12 6DZ
Telephone 01326 231600

www.spiezia.co.uk
Superb organic skin-care products,
herbs and oils, organic calendula
ointment.

The Stamp Collection from Buxton
Foods, 12 Harley Street,
London W1G 9PG
Telephone 020 7637 5505
www.stamp-collection.co.uk
Fabulous range of no-wheat, no-cow's
milk foods. Available from Sainsbury's,
Tesco, Waitrose. ASDA and health food
stores. Website has product information,
recipes and useful links to other sites.

Virani Food Products Ltd.,
10–14 Stewarts Road, Finedon Road
Industrial Estate, Wellingborough,
Northamptonshire NN8 4RJ
Telephone 01933 276483
www.virani.co.uk
Specialist foods including a wide range
of flours suitable for wheat-free and
gluten-free diets.

Viridian Nutrition, 31 Alvis Way,
Royal Oak, Daventry,
Northamptonshire NN11 5PG
Telephone 01327 878050
www.viridian-nutrition.com
Digestive Aid, psyllium, acidophilus
complex, cold-pressed oils, vitamins,
minerals, herbals.

Woodlands Park Dairy, Wimbourne,
Dorset BH21 8LX
Telephone 0120 282 2687
www.woodlands-park.co.uk
sales@woodlands-park.co.uk
Goat's and sheep's milk (plain and fruit)
yoghurts available via health food stores
and major supermarkets.

Xynergy Health Products, Lower Elsted,
Midhurst, West Sussex GU29 0JT
Telephone 01730 813642
Green foods, aloe vera products. Stockist
for Kiwiherb and Manuka products.

Finding a Practitioner

If you live in London, the following multi-therapy centres have a staff of qualified practitioners and offer a wide range of services and valuable information.

The Wren Clinic, All Hallows House, Centre for Natural Health, Idol Lane, London EC3R 5DD
Telephone 020 7283 8908 Monday to Thursday.
www.wrenclinic.co.uk
Nutrition therapy, McTimoney chiropractic, acupuncture, homoeopathy, etc. If you are outside London, All Hallows will try to help you find a practitioner nearer to your home.

Apotheke 20–20, 296 & 300–302 Chiswick High Road, London W2H 1PA
Telephone number for appointments 020 8995 2293
www.apotheke20-20.co.uk
Click Naturopathic Clinic.
Qualified practitioner support also available by telephone to those who cannot travel to London. Personal consultations in London.

What Doctors Don't Tell You,
What Doctors Don't Tell You PLC, 2 Salisbury Road, London, SW19 4EZ
Telephone 0870 444 9886
www.wddty.co.uk
The website of this journal has a very useful Find a Practitioner section.

Candidiasis practitioners,
Jane McWhirter's book *The Practical Guide To Candida* (see page 79) contains a UK directory of practitioners who treat candidiasis with natural medicine.

The Hale Clinic, 7 Park Crescent, London W1B 1PF
Telephone 0870 167 6667
www.haleclinic.com

Health Interlink Ltd., Unit B, Asfordby Business Park, Welby, Melton Mowbray, Leicestershire LE14 3JL
Telephone 01664 810011

www.health-interlink.co.uk
Offers diagnostic/testing services to practitioners for conditions such as candidiasis, parasites, digestive function, intestinal permeability, bacterial overgrowth, food sensitivity and more. The company isn't able to give telephone advice or discuss individual cases but it is happy to tell you if it knows of a practitioner in your area.

Stress The Safeline is primarily for confidential guidance and information on stress. If you're under pressure and want to talk to a qualified therapist or counsellor, or if you're trying to find a practitioner in your local area, try this number.
Telephone 020 7233 5566
Or E-mail ken@chihealthcentres.com

Check with your GP or local Family Health Service Authority (in the phone book) to find out which, if any, alternative and complementary therapies are available through your NHS practice.

The following UK-based organisations hold lists of registered practitioners:

Governing Bodies/Institutes/ Associations of Alternative Medicine, listed at:
www.britishservices.co.uk

British Naturopathic Association, 2 Goswell Road, Street, Somerset BA16 0JG
Telephone 08707 456985
www.naturopaths.org.uk

National Federation of Spiritual Healers, Old Manor Farm Studio, Church Street, Sunbury-on-Thames, Middlesex TW16 6RG
Telephone 0845 123 2777
www.nfsh.org.uk

McTimoney Chiropractic, The McTimoney Chiropractic Association, 21 High Street, Eynsham, Oxford OX8 1HE
Telephone 01865 880974
www.mctimoney-chiropractic.org

The British Chiropractic Association,
17 Blagrave Street, Reading,
Berkshire RG1 1QB
Telephone 0118 950 5950
www.chiropractic-uk.co.uk

General Chiropractic Council,
344–354 Gray's Inn Road,
London WC1X 8BP
Telephone 020 7713 5155
www.gcc-uk.org

The Register of Chinese Herbal Medicine,
www.rchm.org.uk

British Medical Acupuncture Society,
12 Marbury House, Higher Whitley,
Warrington, Cheshire WA4 4QW
Telephone 01925 730727
www.medical-acupuncture.co.uk

The UK Homoeopathic Medical Association, 6 Livingston Road,
Gravesend, Kent DA12 5DZ
Telephone 01474 560336
www.homoeopathy.org

British Homeopathic Association,
15 Clerkenwell Close,
London EC1R 0AA
Telephone 020 7566 7800
www.trusthomeopathy.org.

(Note: when looking for homeopathy websites, be aware of the two different spellings of the word homeopathy/homoeopathy.)

British Complementary Medicine Association, P.O.Box 5122,
Bournemouth, Dorset BH8 0WG
Telephone 0845 345 5977
www.bcma.co.uk

Other Useful Addresses

Digestive Diseases Foundation,
3 St. Andrew's Place, Regents Park,
London NW1 4LB
Telephone 020 7486 0341
www.digestivediseases.org.uk

Hyperactive Children's Support Group (HACSG), 71 Whyke Lane,
Chichester, West Sussex PO19 2LD
www.hacsg.org.uk
Really valuable information for allergy sufferers and for those with allergic and/or hyperactive youngsters. A very dedicated, non-profit-making organisation. Please send large stamped addressed envelope and £1 donation towards expenses.

National Association for Diverticular Disease, 7 Cambridge Road, Orrell,
Wigan, Lancashire WN5 8PL
Telephone 01942 213572
www.ukselfhelp.info/groupNADD.htm

Women's Environmental Network,
P.O.Box 30626, London E1 1TZ
Telephone 020 7481 9004

www.wen.org.uk
For those interested in keeping up to date with environmental issues. Send large stamped addressed envelope for details. Membership available.

Self-Help Website
www.ukselfhelp.info
Click on the alphabet letter you need.

If you are concerned about animal welfare and factory farming and are interested in supporting and receiving information from non-violent pressure groups, contact:

Compassion in World Farming (CIWF), 5A Charles Street, Petersfield,
Hampshire GU32 3EH, England
or CIWF, P.O.Box 206, Cork, Ireland for their Action Pack and membership details. CIWF also have a youth group called FarmWatch.

Farm Animal Welfare Network,
P.O. Box 40, Holmforth, Huddersfield,
West Yorkshire HD7 1QY, England.

Sources of Reference

The Inside Story

Guyton A.C., *Textbook of Medical Physiology*, 8th edition. W.B. Saunders 1991.

Matsen J., *Eating Alive – Prevention Thru Good Digestion*. Crompton Books 1991.

Murray M. and Pizzorno J., *Encyclopaedia of Natural Medicine* Revised, 2nd edition. Little Brown 2000; 126–144.

Smith T. (ed.), *The Human Body*. Dorling Kindersley 1995.

Youngson R., *Royal Society of Medicine Encyclopaedia of Human Health*. Bloomsbury 1995.

What's Up? Acid Reflux

Davies D. and James T.G., 'An investigation into the gastric secretion of a hundred normal persons over the age of sixty', *British Medical Journal* 1930;i:1–14.

Dethlefsen T. and Dahlke R., *The Healing Power of Illness*. Element 1994:133.

Graham D.Y. et al., 'Why do apparently healthy people use antacid tablets?' *American Journal of Gastroenterology* 1983;78:257–260.

Murray M.T., 'Indigestion'. *Encyclopedia of Nutritional Supplements*, Prima 1996;461–462.

Report. 'When heartburn goes from "nuisance" to "dangerous"'. *Tufts University Diet & Nutrition Letter* 1996;14[6]6:4–5.

Sturnilio G.C. et al., 'Inhibition of gastric acid secretion reduces zinc absorption in man', *Journal of the American College of Nutrition* 1991;4:372–375.

Vogel H.C.A., *The Nature Doctor*. Mainstream Publishing 1989;448–450.

What's Up? Bloating and Gas

Sanders M.E. et al., 'Performance of commercial cultures in fluid milk applications', *Journal of Dairy Science* 1996;79:943–955.

Schiffrin E.J, et al., 'Immunomodulation of human blood cells following the ingestion of lactic acid bacteria', *Journal of Dairy Science* 1995;78:491–497.

What's Up? Candida

Bauman D.S and Hagglund H.E., 'Correlation between certain polysystem chronic complaints and an enzyme immunoassay with antigens of *Candida albicans*', *Journal of the Advancement of Medicine* 1991;4:5–19.

Boero M. et al., 'Candida overgrowth in gastric juice of peptic ulcer subjects on short- and long-term treatment with H2 receptor antagonists', *Digestion* 1983;28:158–163.

Chapdelaine P.A. et al., 'Candidiasis', *Townsend Letter for Doctors* 1995;138:64–75.

Crook W.G., *The Yeast Connection*, 2nd edition. Jackson T.N. Professional Books 1984.

Crook W.G., *The Yeast Connection and the Woman*. Jackson T.N. Professional Books 1995.

Eaton K.K., 'Gut fermentation: a reappraisal of an old clinical condition, diagnostic tests and management. A discussion paper', *Journal of the Royal Society of Medicine* 1991;ii:669–71.

Hunnisett A. et al., 'Gut fermentation or the autobrewery syndrome: a new clinical test with initial observations and discussions of clinical and biochemical conditions', *Journal of Nutritional Medicine* 1990;1:33–39.

Iwata K., 'Toxins produced by *Candida albicans*', *Contributions to Microbiology and Immunology* 1977;4:77–85.

Kaneda Y. et al., 'In vitro effects of berberine sulphate on the growth of *Entamoeba histolytica*, *Giardia lamblia* and *Trichomonas vaginalis*', Annals of Tropical Medicine and Parasitology 1991;85:417–425.

Moore G.S. and Atkins R.D., 'The fungicidal and fungistatic effects of an aqueous garlic extract on medically important yeast-like fungi', *Mycologia* 1977;69:341–348.

Murray M.T., 'Candidiasis', *Encyclopedia of Nutritional Supplements*, Prima 1996;432–433.

Rubinstein E. et al., 'Antibacterial activity of the pancreatic fluid', *Gastroenterology* 1985; 88:927–932.

Russo A. et al., 'The effect of acute hyperglycemia on small intestinal motility in normal subjects', *Diabetologia* 1996; 39:984–989.

Shahani K.M. and Friend B.A., 'Nutritional and therapeutic aspects of lactobacilli', *Journal of Applied Nutrition* 1984;36:125–152.

Stiles J.C. et al., 'The inhibition of *Candida albicans* by oregano', *Journal of Applied Nutrition* 1995;47:96–102.

Woodhead M., 'Antibiotic resistance', *British Journal of Hospital Medicine* 1996;56:314–315.

What's Up? Constipation

Marsden K., 'Constipation – how to keep going', *Townsend Letter for Doctors* January 1993;114:107–109.

Page, Christine R., *Frontiers of Health*. C.W. Daniel 1992:123–124.

Passmore A.P. and Wilson-Davies K. et al., 'A comparison of Agiolax (senna & fibre) and lactulose in elderly patients with chronic constipation', *Pharmacology* 1993; 47[1]:249–52.

Robbins, J., *Diet For a New America*. 1987:258 & 260.

What's Up? Diarrhoea?

Babb R.R., 'Coffee, sugars and chronic diarrhoea', *Postgraduate Medicine* 1984;75:82–87.

Barness L.A., 'Safety considerations with high ascorbic acid dosage', *Annals of the New York Academy of Sciences* 1975;258:523–528. Photocopy of review.

Colombel J.F. et al., 'Bifidobacterium longum reduces erythromycin-induced gastrointestinal effects', *Lancet* 1987;ii:43.

Eherer A.H. et al., 'Effect of psyllium, calcium polycarbophil and wheat bran on secretory diarrhoes induced by phenolphthalein', *Gastroenterology* 1993;104:1007–1012.

Hyams J.S. et al., 'Carbohydrate malabsorption following fruit juice ingestion in young children', *Pediatrics* 1988;82:64–68.

James J.M. and Burks A.W., 'Food-associated gastrointestinal disease', *Current Opinion in Pediatrics* 1996;8:471–475. Photocopy of review.

Khin-Maung U. et al., 'Clinical trial of berberine in acute watery diarrhoea', *British Medical Journal* 1985;291:1601–1605.

Montes R.G and Perman J.A., 'Lactose Intolerance', *Postgraduate Medicine* 1991; 89:175–184.

Murray M.T., *The Healing Power of Herbs. Goldenseal and other berberine-containing plants*, 2nd edition. Prima. 1995;162–172.

Murray M.T., *The Healing Power of Herbs. Green tea*, 2nd edition. Prima. 1995;192–196

What's Up? Food Allergies

Anderson I.H., Levine A.S. and Levitt M.D., 'Incomplete absorption of the carbohydrate in all purpose wheat flour', *New England Journal of Medicine* 1981;304:891–892.

Andre F. et al., 'Role of new allergens and of allergens consumption in the increased incidence of food sensitizations in France', *Toxicology* 1994;93:77–83.

Article: 'Are you sure it's a food allergy?' Reported in *Tufts University Diet & Nutrition Letter* 1993;10[12]:2&7.

Bachert C. et al., 'Decreased reactivity in allergic rhinitis after intravenous application of calcium. A study on the alteration of local airway resistance after nasal allergen provocation', *Arzneimittelforsch* 1990; 40:984–987.

Bjarnason I., Peters T.J. and Levi J., 'Intestinal permeability: clinical correlates', *Digestive Diseases* 1986;4:83–92.

Bland J., 'The food for one may be poison for another', *International Journal of Alternative and Complementary Medicine* 1995;13[3]:16–17.

Collins A.M. et al., 'Bovine milk, including pasteurized milk, contains antibodies directed against allergens of clinical importance to man', *International Archives of Allergy and Applied Immunology* 1991;96:362–367.

Cooper B.T., Holmes G.K.T., Ferguson R.A., Thompson R.N.A. and Cooke W.T., 'Gluten-sensitive diarrhoea without evidence of coeliac disease', *Gastroenterology* 1980; 79:801–806.

Cummings W.A. and Williams E.W., 'Transport of large breakdown products of dietary protein through the gut wall', *Gut* 1978; 19:715.

Fan Y.Y. and Chapkin R.S., 'Peritoneal macrophage prostaglandin E1 synthesis is altered by dietary gamma-linolenic acid', *Journal of Nutrition* 1994;122[8]:1600–1606.

Gerrard J.W. et al., 'The familial incidence of allergic disease', *Annals of Allergy* 1976;36:10.

Hadjivassiliou M., Gibson A., Davies-Jones G.A.B., Lobo A.J., Stephenson T.J. and Milford-Ward A., 'Does cryptic gluten sensitivity play a part in neurological illness?' *Lancet* 1996;347:369–371.

Henzgen M. et al., 'Food hypersensitivity in patients with tree pollen allergy and the influence of hyposensitization', *Allergologie* 1991;14[3]:90–94.

Laino C., '*H. pylori* implicated in allergies', *Medical Tribune* March 1994: 1.

Lipski E., *Digestive Wellness*, 2nd edition. Keats Publishing 2000;331–332.

Metcalfe D., 'Food hypersensitivity', *Journal of Allergy and Clinical Immunology* 1984;73:749–761.

Middleton E. et al., 'Naturally occurring flavonoids and human basophil histamine release', *Archives of Allergy and Applied Immunology* 1985;77:155–157.

Minor J.D. et al., 'Leukocyte inhibition factor in delayed-onset food sensitivity', *Journal of Allergy and Clinical Immunology* 1980;6:314.

Murray M. and Pizzorno J., *Encyclopaedia of Natural Medicine*, Revised 2nd edition. Little Brown 2000;464–475.

Murray M.T., Food Allergy. *Encyclopedia of Nutritional Supplements*. Prima 1996; 448–449.

Randolph, T.G. and Moss, R. W., *Allergies – Your Hidden Enemy*. Thorsons; 49–63, 69–93, 178–187, 215–222.

Rinkel R.J., 'Food allergy iv: the function and clinical application of the Rotary Diversified Diet', *Journal of Pediatrics* 1948;32:266.

Sampson H.A, Broadbent K.R. and Bernhisel-Broadbent J., 'Spontaneous release of histamine from basophils and histamine-releasing factor in patients with atopic dermatitis and food hypersensitivity', *New England Journal of Medicine* 1989;321:228–232.

Sampson H.A., 'Food hypersensitivity and dietary management in atopic dermatitis', *Pediatric Dermatology* 1992;9:376–379.

Schoenthaler S.J., Doraz W.E. and Wakefield J.A., 'The impact of a low food additive and sucrose diet on academic performance in 803 New York City public schools', *International Journal of Biosocial Research* 1986; 8[2]:185–195.

Trevino R.J., 'Immunologic mechanisms in the production of food sensitivities', *Laryngoscope* 1981;91:1913.

Walker R. and Quattrucci E., Nutritional and toxicological aspects of food processing. (Taylor & Francis, Philadelphia).

Walker-Smith J.A., 'Food sensitive enteropathies', *Clinics in Gastroenterology* 1986;15[1]:55–69.

Weir M.R. et al., 'Depression of vitamin B6 levels due to theophylline', *Annals of Allergy* 1990;65:59–62.

Young E. et al., 'A population study of food intolerance', *Lancet* 1994;343:127–129.

What's Up? Gallstones

Baggio G. et al., 'Olive oil enriched diet: effect on serum lipoprotein levels and biliary cholesterol saturation', *American Journal of Clinical Nutrition* 1988;47:960–964.

Breneman J.C., 'Allergy elimination diet as the most effective gallbladder diet', *Annals of Allergy* 1968;26:83–87.

Capper W.M et al., 'GALLSTONES, gastric secretion and flatulent dyspepsia', *Lancet* 1967;i:413–415.

De Muro P. and Fiscari A., 'Experimental studies on allergic cholecystitis', *Gastroenterology* 1946;6:302–314.

Douglas B.R. et al., 'Coffee stimulation of cholecystokinin release and gallbladder contraction in humans', *American Journal of Clinical Nutrition* 1990;52:553–556.

Everhart J.E., 'Contributions of obesity and weight loss to gallstone disease', *Annals of Internal Medicine* 1993;119:1029–1035.

Gustaffson U. et al., 'The effect of vitamin C in high doses on plasma and biliary lipid composition in patients with cholesterol gallstones: prolongation of the nucleation time', *European Journal of Clinical Investigation* 1997;27:387–391.

Heaton K.W., et al., 'An explanation for gallstones in normal weight women: slow intestinal transit', *Lancet* 1993;341:8–10.

Jayanthi V., Malathi S., Ramathilakam B., et al., 'Is the vegetarianism a precipitating factor for gallstones in cirrhotics? *Tropical Gastroenterology* 1998;19:21–23.

Jenkins S.A., 'Vitamin C and gallstone formation: a preliminary report', *Experentia* 1977;33:1616–1617.

Kamrath R.O. et al., 'Cholelithiasis in patients treated with a very low calorie diet', *American Journal of Clinical Nutrition* 1992; 56: 2558–2578.

Lee D.W.T., Gilmore C.J., Bonorris G., et al., 'Effect of dietary cholesterol on biliary lipids in patients with gallstones and normal subjects', *American Journal of Clinical Nutrition* 1985;42:414.

Maclure K.M., et al., 'Weight, diet, and the risk of symptomatic and gallstones in middle-aged women', *New England Journal of Medicine* 1989;321:563–569.

Marks J.W. et al., 'Lack of correlation between serum lipoproteins and biliary cholesterol saturation in patients with gallstones', *Digestive Diseases and Sciences* 1984; 29:1118–1122.

Moerman C.J. et al., 'Dietary risk factors for clinically diagnosed gallstones in middle-aged men: a 25 year follow-up study/The Zutphen Study', *Annals of Epidemiology* 1994; 4:248–254.

Murray M. and Pizzorno J., *Encyclopaedia of Natural Medicine*, revised 2nd edition 2002; 484, 479.

Murray M.T., *Gallstones. Encyclopedia of Nutritional Supplements*. Prima 1996;449–450.

Murray M.T., *Milk Thistle. The Healing Power of Herbs*, 2nd edition. Prima 1995;243–252.

Necheles H. et al., 'Allergy of the gallbladder', *American Journal of Digestive Diseases* 1949; 7:238–241.

Nervi F. et al., 'Influence of legume intake on biliary lipids and cholesterol saturation in young Chilean men', *Gastroenterology* 1989;96:825–830.

Pacel S., 'Sunbathing and gallstones', *Lancet* 1992;339:241.

Petitti D.B. et al., 'Association of a history of gallbladder disease with a reduced concentration of high-density lipoprotein cholesterol', *New England Journal of Medicine* 1981;304:1396–1398.

Pixley F. and Mann J., 'Dietary factors in the aetiology of gallstones: a case control study', *Gut* 1988; 29:1511–1515.

Pixley F. et al., 'Effect of vegetarianiam on development of gallstones in women', *British Medical Journal* 1985;291:11–22.

Sarles H. et al., 'Diet and cholesterol gallstones', *Digestion* 1978;17:121–127.

Simon J.A., Grady D., Snabes M.C. et al., 'Ascorbic acid supplement use and the prevalence of gallbladder disease', *Journal of*

Clinical Epidemiology 1998;51:257–265.

Simon J.A., 'Ascorbic acid and cholesterol gallstones', *Medical Hypotheses* 1993; 40:81–84.

Somerville K.W. et al., 'Stones in the common bile duct: experience with medical dissolution therapy', *Postgraduate Medicine* 1985; 61:313–316.

Spirit B.A. et al., 'Gallstone formation in obese women treated by a low calorie diet', *International Journal of Obesity* 1995; 19:593–595.

Stampfer M.J. et al., 'Risk of symptomatic gallstones in women with severe obesity', *American Journal of Clinical Nutrition* 1992; 55:652–658.

Tandon R.K. et al., 'Dietary habits of gallstone patients in Northern India: a case control study', *Journal of Clinical Gastroenterology* 1996;22:23–27.

Thornton J.R., Heaton K. and MacFarland D.G., 'A relation between high density lipoprotein cholesterol and bile cholesterol saturation', *Lancet* 1981;i:1352–1354.

Toouli J., Jablonski P. and Watts J., 'Gallstone dissolution in man using cholic acid and lecithin', *Lancet* 1975;ii:1124–1126.

Trowell H., Burkitt D. and Heaton K., Dietary fibre, fibre-depleted foods, and disease. *New York Academic Press* 1985;289–304.

Tuzhilin S.A. et al., 'The treatment of patients with gallstones by lecithin', *American Journal of Gastroenterology* 1976;165:231–35.

Weisberg H.F., 'Pathogenesis of gallstones', *Annals of Clinical and Laboratory Science* 1984;14:243–251.

What's Up? Haemorrhoids/Piles

Moesgaard F. et al., 'High fiber diet reduces bleeding and pain in patients with hemorrhoids', *Diseases of the Colon and Rectum* 1982;82:454–456.

Murray M. and Pizzorno J., *Encyclopaedia of Natural Medicine*, Revised 2nd edition. Little Brown 2002;510.

Murray M.T., *Flavonoids. Encyclopedia of Nutritional Supplements*. Prima 1996;320–331.

Page, C.R., *Frontiers of Health*. C. W. Daniel 1992;123–124.

Webster D.J. et al., 'The use of bulk evacuation in patients with hemmorhoids', *British Journal of Surgery* 1978;65:291–292.

What's Up? Intestinal Parasites

Choudry V.P., Sabir M. and Bhide V.N., 'Berberine in giardiasis', *Indian Pediatrics* 1972;9:143–146.

Kaneda Y. et al., 'In vitro effects of berberine sulphate on the growth of *Entamoeba histolytica, Giardia lamblia* and *Trichomonas vaginalis'*, *Annals of Tropical Medicine and Parasitology* 1991;85:417–425.

Mirelman D., Monheit D. and Varon S., 'Inhibition of growth of *Entamoeba histolytica* by allicin, the active principle of garlic extract (*Allium sativum*)', *Journal of Infectious Diseases* 1987;156:243–244.

Murray M. and Pizzorno J., *Encyclopaedia of Natural Medicine*, Revised 2nd edition. Little Brown 2000;436–437.

Murray M.T., 'Goldenseal and other berberine-containing plants'. *The Healing Power of Herbs*, 2nd edition. Prima 1995; 162–172

What's Up? Irritable Bowel Syndrome

Arffmann S. et al., 'The effect of coarse wheat bran in the irritable bowel syndrome. A double-blind crossover study', *Scandinavian Journal of Gastroenterology* 1985;20:295–298.

Barton J.R., 'Investigation and surgery in IBS – a cautionary series', *Scottish Medical Journal* 1994;39:80–81.

Bentley S.J. et al., 'Food hypersensitivity in irritable bowel syndrome', *Lancet* 1983; ii:295–297.

Blanchard E.B. et al., 'Relaxation training as a treatment for irritable bowel syndrome', *Biofeedback Self Regulation* 1993;18:125–132.

Bohmer C.J. and Tuynman H.A., 'The clinical relevance of lactose malabsorption in irritable bowel syndrome', *European Journal of Gastroenterology and Hepatology* 1996; 8:1013–1016.

Danilewitz M., 'Irritable bowel syndrome: eight questions physicians often ask', *The Consultant* 1991;50–52.

Editorial. 'Dietary fibre, food intolerance and irritable bowel syndrome,' *Nutrition Review* 1990; 48[9]:343–346.

Farah D.A. et al., 'Specific food intolerance: its place as a cause of gastrointestinal symptoms', *Gut* 1985;26:164–168.

Fernandez-Banares F. et al., 'Sugar malabsorption in functional bowel disease: clinical implications', *American Journal of Gastroenterology* 1993;88:2044–2050.

Fielding J. and Kehoe M., 'Different dietary fibre formulations and the irritable bowel syndrome', *Irish Journal of Medical Science* 1984;153: 178–180.

Fielding J., 'Detailed history and examination assist positive clinical diagnosis of the irritable bowel syndrome', *Journal of Clinical Gastroenterology* 1983;5:495–497

Francis C.Y., 'Bran and IBS: time for reappraisal', *Lancet* 1994;344:39–40.

Gay L., 'Mucous colitis complicated by colonic polyposis, relieved by allergy management',

American Journal Digestive Diseases 1937; 3:326–329.

Gertner D. and Powell-Tuck J., 'Irritable bowel sydrome and food intolerance', *Practitioner* 1994;238:499–504.

Goldsmith G. and Levin J.S., 'Effect of sleep quality on symptoms of irritable bowel syndrome', *Digestive Diseases and Sciences* 1993;38:1809–1814.

Guillory G., *IBS: A Doctor's Plan for Chronic Digestive Troubles*. Hartley & Marks; 114–138.

Hollander E., 'Mucous colitis due to food allergy', *American Journal of Medical Science* 1927;174:495–500.

Jones V. et al., 'Food intolerance: a major factor in the pathogenesis of irritable bowel syndrome', *Lancet* 1982;ii:1115–1118.

King T.S. et al., 'Abnormal colonic fermentation in irritable bowel syndrome', *Lancet* 1998; 352:1187–1189.

Lewis P.J., 'Irritable bowel syndrome: emotional factors and acupuncture treatment', *Journal of Chinese Medicine* 1992; 40:9–12.

Lin M. et al., 'Influence of nonfermented dairy products containing bacterial starter cultrures on lactose maldigestion in humans', *Journal of Dairy Science* 1991;74:87–95.

Lininger S.W., Gaby A.R., Austin S., Brown D. J., Wright J.V. and Duncan A., The Natural Pharmacy. Prima 1999;109–110.

Longstreth G.F., 'Irritable bowel syndrome: a multi billion dollar-problem', *Gastroenterology* 1995:109 2029–2042.

Lucey M.R. et al., 'Is bran efficacious in irritable bowel syndrome? A double-blind placebo controlled crossover study', *Gut* 1987; 28:221–225.

Manning A.P. et al., 'Wheat fibre and irritable bowel syndrome', *Lancet* 1977;2:417–418.

Murray M. and Pizzorno J., *Encyclopaedia of Natural Medicine*, Revised 2nd edition. Little Brown 2000; 609–613.

Nanda R. et al., 'Food intolerance and the irritable bowel syndrome', *Gut* 1989;30: 1099–1104.

Narducci F., Snape W., Battle W., Lodon R. and Cohen S., 'Increasd colonic motility during exposure to a stressful situation', *Digestive Diseases and Sciences* 1985;30:40–44.

Nash P. et al., 'Peppermint oil does not relieve the pain of irritable bowel syndrome', *British Journal of Clinical Practice* 1986;40:292–293.

Petitpierre, M., Gumowski P. and Girard J., 'Irritable bowel syndrome and hypersensitivity to food', *Annals of Allergy* 1985;54:538–540.

Rees W. et al., 'Treating irritable bowel syndrome with peppermint oil', *British Medical Journal* 1979;ii:835–836.

Rogers, S.A., 'Environmental medicine: the fibromyalgia fiasco', *Townsend Letter for Doctors* 1995;141:62.

Russo A., Fraser R. and Horowitz M., 'The effect of acute hyperglycaemia on small intestinal motility in normal subjects', *Diabetologia* 1996;39:984–989.

Ryan W., Kelly M. and Fielding J., 'The normal personality profile of irritable bowel syndrome patients', *Irish Journal of Medical Science* 1984;153:127–129.

Shaw G. et al., 'Stress management for irritable bowel syndrome: a controlled trial', *Digestion* 1991;50:36–42.

Smith M.A. et al., 'Food intolerance, atrophy and irritable bowel syndrome', *Lancet* 1985; 2:1064.

Soloft J. et al., 'A double-blind trial of the effect of wheat bran on symptoms of irritable bowel syndrome', *Lancet* 1976;i:270–273.

Somerville K. et al., 'Delayed release peppermint oil capsules (Colpermin) for the spastic colon syndrome: a pharmacokinetic study', *British Journal of Clinical Pharmacology* 1984;18:638–640.

Svedlund J., Sjodin I., Doteval G. and Gillberg R., 'Upper gastrointestinal and mental symptoms in the irritable bowel syndrome', *Scandinavian Journal of Gastroenterology* 1985; 20: 595–601.

Walker A. et al., 'Artichoke leaf extract reduces symptoms of irritable bowel syndrome in a post-marketing surveillance study', *Phytotherapy Research* 2001;15:58–61.

Werbach, M.R., *Nutritional Influences on Illness: Irritable Bowel Syndrome*. Thorsons;274–277.

Weser E., Rubin W., Ross L. and Sleisenger M.H., 'Lactase deficiency in patients with irritable colon syndrome', *New England Journal of Medicine* 1965;273:1070–1075.

Zwetchkenbaum J. and Burakoff R., 'The irritable bowel syndrome and food hypersensitivity', *Annals of Allergy* 1988;61:47–49.

What's Up? Lactose Intolerance

Baer D., 'Lactase deficiency and yoghurt', *Social Biology* 1970;17:143.

Bayless T.M. and Rosenweig N.S., 'A racial difference in incidence of lactase deficiency: a survey of milk intolerance and lactase deficiency in healthy adult males', *Journal of the American Medical Association* 1966; 197[12]:968–972.

Bayless T.M., Rothfeld B., Massa C., Wise L., Paige D. and Bedine M.S., 'Lactose and milk intolerance: clinical implications', *New England Journal of Medicine* 1975; 292:1156–1159.

Bhatia S.J., Kochar N., Abraham P., Nair N.G.

and Mehta A.P., 'Lactobacillus acidophilus inhibits growth of Campylobacter pylori in vitro', Journal of Clinical Microbiology 1989; 27[10]:2328–2330.

Colombel J.F. et al., 'Yoghurt with Bifidobacterium longum reduces erythromycin induced gastrointestinal effects', Lancet 1987;2:43.

Editorial. 'Marketers milk misconceptions on lactose intolerance', Tufts University Diet & Nutrition Letter 1995;12[10]:4–7.

Fernandes C.F., Shahani K.M. and Amer M.A., 'Therapeutic role of dietary lactobacilli and lactobacillic fermented dairy products', Federation of European Microbiological Societies Microbiology Review 1987;46:343–356.

Friend B.A. and Shahani K.M., 'Nutritional and therapeutic aspects of lactobacilli', Journal of Applied Nutrition 1984;2:125–153.

Gallagher C.R., Molleson A.L. and Caldwell J.H., 'Lactose intolerance and fermented dairy products', Journal of the American Dietetic Association 1974;65:418–419.

Gilliland S.E. and Speck M.L., 'Antagonistic action of Lactobacillus acidophilus towards intestinal and foodborne pathogens in associative cultures', Journal of Food Protection 1977;40[12]:820–823.

Golden B.R. and Gorbach S.L., 'The effect of milk and Lactobacillus feeding on human intestinal bacterial enzyme activity', American Journal of Clinical Nutrition 1984;39:756–761.

Gorbach S.L., 'Lactic acid bacteria and human health', Annals of Medicine 1990;22:37–41.

Kim H.S. and Gilliland S.E., 'Lactobacillus acidophilus as a dietary adjunct for milk to aid lactose digestion in humans', Journal of Dairy Science 1983;66:959–966.

Montes R.G. and Perman J.A., 'Lactose intolerance', Postgraduate Medicine 1991; 89:175–184.

Reasoner J., Maculan T.P., Rand A.G. and Thayer W.R., 'Clinical studies with low lactose milk', American Journal of Clinical Nutrition 1981;34:54–60.

Report. 'If you think you can't stomach milk…' Tufts University Diet & Nutrition Letter 1995;13[7]:7–8.

Skala I., Larnacora V. and Pirk F., 'Lactose-free milk as a solution of problems associated with dietetic treatment of lactose intolerance', Digestion 1971;4:326–332.

Weser E., Rubin W., Ross L. and Sleisenger M.H., 'Lactase deficiency in patients with irritable colon syndrome', New England Journal of Medicine 1965;273:1070–1075.

Weser E. and Sleisenger M.H., 'Lactosuria and lactase deficiency in adult coeliac disease', Gastroenterology 1965;48:571–578.

Zeigler E.E., Fomon S.J., Nelson S.E., Rebouche C.J. and Edwards B.B. et al., 'Cow's milk feeding in infancy: further observations on blood loss from the gastrointestinal tract', Journal of Paediatrics 1990;116:11–18.

What's Up? Leaky Gut Syndrome

Bjarnason I., Peters T.J. and Levi A.J., 'Intestinal permeability: clinical correlates', Digestive Diseases 1986;4:83–92.

Cummings W.A. and Williams E.W., 'Transport of large breakdown products of dietary protein through the gut wall', Gut 1978; 19:715.

Hunnisett A. et al., 'Gut fermentation (or the auto-brewery) syndrome', Journal of Nutritional Medicine 1990;1[1]:33–38.

King C.E. and Toskes P., 'Small intestine bacterial overgrowth', Gastroenterology 1979; 76:1035–1055.

Matthews G., 'Gut fermentation', Journal of the Royal Society of Medicine 1992;58:305.

What's Up? Ulcers

Beil W. et al., 'Effects of flavonoids on parietal cell acid secretion, gastric mucosal prostaglandin production and Helicobacter pylori growth', Arzneim Forsch 1995; 45:697–700.

Berstad K. and Berstad A., 'Helicobacter pylori infection in peptic ulcer disease', Scandinavian Journal of Gastroenterology 1993;28:561–567.

Bhatia S.J., Kochar N., Abraham P., Nair N.G. and Mehta A.P., 'Lactobacillus acidophilus inhibits growth of Campylobacter pylori in vitro', Journal of Clinical Microbiology 1989; 27[10]:2328–2330.

Cater R.E., 'Helicobacter pylori (also known as Campylobacter pylori) as the major causal factor in chronic hypochlorhydria', Medical Hypotheses 1992;39:367–374.

Click L., 'Deglycyrrhizinated liquorice in peptic ulcer', Lancet 1982;2:817.

Dethlefsen T. and Dahlke R., The Healing Power of Illness. Element 1994:133–134.

Feldman E.J. et al., 'Stress and peptic ulcer disease', Gastroenterology 1980;78:1087–1089.

Gershon M.D., The Second Brain. HarperPerennial 1999:105–108.

Hay, L., You Can Heal Your Life. Eden Grove 1984:134.

Howden C.V. et al., 'Relationship between gastric secretion and infection', Gut 1987;28:96–107.

Kumar N. et al., 'Effect of milk on patients with duodenal ulcers', British Medical Journal 1986;293:666.

Marshall B.J. et al., 'Bismuth sub-salicylate suppression of Helicobacter pylori in non-ulcer dyspepsia: a double-blind placebo-controlled trial', *Digestive Diseases & Sciences* 1993;38:1674–1680.

Murray M.T., Licorice. *The Healing Power of Herbs*, 2nd edition. Prima 1995;228–239.

Murray M.T., Flavonoids. *Encyclopedia of Nutritional Supplements*. Prima 1996;320–331.

Murray M.T., Ulcers. *Encyclopedia of Nutritional Supplements*. Prima 1996;486–487.

Page, C. R., *Frontiers of Health*. C. W. Daniel 1992;164–165.

Rydning A. et al., 'Prophylactic effects of dietary fibre in duodenal ulcer disease', *Lancet* 1982; 2:736–739.

Thomson M.A. et al., 'Canine-human transmission of Gastrospirillum hominis', *Lancet* 1994;343:1605–1606.

Transcript of Horizon documentary *Ulcer Wars*. BBC television. First transmitted 16 May 1994.

Van Marle J. et al., 'Deglcyrrhizinised liquorice and the renewal of rat stomach epithelium', *European Journal of Pharmacology* 1981; 72:219–225.

Vogel H.C.A., *The Nature Doctor*. Mainstream Publishing 1989;497.

Weil J. et al., 'Prophylactic aspirin and risk of peptic ulcer bleeding', *British Medical Journal* 1995;310:827–830.

Essential Extras: Fibre Tips

Francis C.Y. and Whorwell P.J., 'Bran and the irritable bowel syndrome: time for reappraisal', *Lancet* 1994;344:19–24.

Passmore A.P. and Wilson-Davies K. et al., 'A comparison of Agiolax (senna & fibre) and lactulose in elderly patients with chronic constipation', *Pharmacology* 1993; 47[1]:249–52.

Robbins, J., *Diet For a New America* 1987; 284–285.

Thompson W.C.T., 'Doubts about bran', *Lancet* 1994;344:3.

Wason H.S. et al., 'Fibre supplemented food may damage your health', *Lancet* 1996; 348:319–320.

Essential Extras: Probiotics

Amin A.H. et al., 'Berberine sulphate: antimicrobial activity, bioassay and mode of action', *Canadian Journal of Microbiology* 1969; 15:1067–1076.

Bengmark S., 'Ecological control of the gastrointestinal tract – the role of probiotic flora', *Gut* 42:2–7.

Bhatia S.J., Kochar N., Abraham P., Nair N.G. and Mehta A.P., '*Lactobacillus acidophilus* inhibits growth of *Campylobacter pylori* in vitro', *Journal of Clinical Microbiology* 1989; 27[10]:2328–2330.

Black F. et al., 'Effect of lactic acid producing bacteria on the human intestinal microflora during Ampicillin treatment', *Scandinavian Journal of Infectious Diseases* 1991;23:247–254.

Black F.T. et al., 'Prophylactic efficacy of lactobacilli on traveller's diarrhoea', *Travel Medicine* 1989;333–335.

Gilliland S.E. and Speck M.L., 'Antagonistic action of *Lactobacillus acidophilus* towards intestinal and foodborne pathogens in associative cultures', *Journal of Food Protection* 1977;40[12]:820–823.

Gottschall, E., *Food and the Gut Reaction*. The Kirkton Press; 21–41.

King C.E. and Toskes P., 'Small intestine bacterial overgrowth', *Gastroenterology* 1979; 76:1035–1055.

Metchnikoff E., *The Prolongation of Life*. Arna Press, New York 1908. Reprinted photocopy.

Mogensen G., 'Health properties of *Lactobacillus acidophilus* LA-5™ and *Bifidobacterium lactis* BB-12™ in a probiotic or functional food concept', edited article dated March 1998.

Plummer, N., *The Lactic Acid Bacteria – Their Role in Human Health*. Bio-Med Publications, no date.

Rubinstein E. et al., 'Antibacterial activity of the pancreatic fluid', *Gastroenterology* 1985; 88:927–932.

Schriffin E.J. et al., 'Immunomodulation of human blood cells following the ingestions of lactic acid bacteria', *Journal of Dairy Science* 1995;78:491–497.

Sun D. et al., 'Berberine sulphate blocks adherence of *Streptococcus pyogenes* to epithelial cells, fibronectin and headecane', *Antimicrobial Agents and Chemotherapy* 1988;32(9);1370–1374.

Essential Extras: Digestion and Stress

Bhattacharya S.K. and Mitra S.K., 'Anxiolytic activity of panax ginseng roots: an experimental study', *Journal of Ethnopharmacology* 1991;34:87–92.

Chou T., 'Wake up and smell the coffee: caffeine, coffee and the medical consequences', *Western Journal of Medicine* 1992;157:544–553.

Farnsworth N.R. et al., 'Siberian ginseng (*Eleutherococcus senticosus*): current status as an adaptogen', *Economic and Medicinal Plant Research* 1985;1:156–215.

Murray M.T., *Panax Ginseng. The Healing Power of Herbs*, 2nd edition. Prima 1995;265–279.

Murray M.T., Anxiety. *Encyclopedia of Nutritional Supplements*, Prima 1996;424.

Index